Y0-BYN-409

LA JOLLA CANCER RESEARCH FOUNDATION

The Miracle on Torrey Pines Mesa

by

William H. Fishman, Ph.D., M.D. hc

Founder and President Emeritus,
La Jolla Cancer Research Foundation

La Jolla Cancer Research Foundation

Library of Congress Catalogue Card Number 95-81189

All rights reserved. No part of this publication may be reproduced, stored in a retrieval system, or transmitted, in any form or by any means, electronic, mechanical, photocopying, recording or otherwise, without prior permission of the copyright owner.

© La Jolla Cancer Research Foundation, La Jolla, 1995
ISBN 0-9647206-0-4

DEDICATION AND ACKNOWLEDGEMENTS

Dedicated to the memory of our parents, Abe and Goldie Fishman and Charles and Ethel Waterman. Our deepest thanks goes to the efforts of my co-workers (listed on pages 214 and 215) over 5 decades.

The Fannie E. Rippel Foundation sponsorship and support of this volume is most appreciated. The Rippel Foundation was a sponsor of the publication in 1976 of "Oncodevelopmental Gene Expression" by Academic Press. That volume contained the papers presented at the San Diego meeting of the International Group for the Study of Carcinoembryonic Proteins. This was the progenitor of the International Society for Oncodevelopmental Biology and Medicine, established in Marburg in 1978.

Sincere thanks are expressed to Lillian Fishman for her valuable editorial suggestions, to Wendy Sunday for word-processing this manuscript and its many revisions and to Muizz Hasham, Manager, Biomedical Photography/ Graphics for preparing the camera ready art.

We appreciate receiving permission from Richard Gabriel Chase, artist, to reproduce his oil painting on the dust cover and from Alice di Gesu, to print the photo by her late husband, Antony, of Bill & Lil Fishman.

TABLE OF CONTENTS

FOREWORDS
This book has two forewords, one by
Professor William J. McGill and the other by
Professor Sidney Weinhouse.

Foreword by William J. McGill,
President Emeritus, Columbia University

This is an unusual personal memoir describing the life and times of Dr. William H. Fishman: scientist and cancer research pioneer.

It begins at the beginning with the emigration of his parents from a suburb of Odessa in the Ukraine to homestead in central Canada in 1908, six years prior to his birth. The personal story ends with the construction of a remarkable, independent cancer research laboratory in La Jolla, California. Dr. Fishman built it, made it famous, and then turned it over to his chosen successors on his retirement in 1989.

The fifty years between Bill Fishman's Ph.D. in Biochemistry and his retirement witnessed an amazing transformation in the field. He entered graduate school at the University of Toronto in 1935 and earned his Ph.D. in 1939. In Toronto, while a student, he began to work on an enzyme, beta-glucuronidase. There was no inkling that it would later play a crucial role in his career. In 1939, he married Lillian Waterman with absolutely no doubt about how important that step would become. Their life-partnership began when she went to work in his laboratory and set out to type his doctoral dissertation. It continues undiminished at this writing, 56 years later.

All these formative events and everything else that happened afterwards are chronicled in Dr. Fishman's account. It is difficult to believe that when he started out in the mid-1930s, biochemistry and cancer research were not considered entirely respectable by senior scientists in biology and chemistry. These fields have been completely transformed in Dr. Fishman's lifetime, in no small measure because of his work.

When Fishman was a young Assistant Professor at the University of Chicago in 1946, he and Dr. A. John Anlyan discovered that high levels of the enzyme beta-glucuronidase are present in cancerous tissue. The result was totally unexpected; at variance with what was then widely believed.

The discovery made Bill Fishman's scientific reputation. It also changed biochemistry fundamentally because it was among the earliest reports of an enzyme as a tumor marker. From then on young Dr. Fishman was in cancer research, and biochemistry was seen increasingly as a crucial tool for cancer study.

Out of this chance observation, for which his native brilliance and early hard work had been preparing him all his life, there emerged an entirely new field of medicine, oncodevelopmental biology. It produced a series of remarkable papers and led eventually to the development of one of the first cancer centers at Tufts University Schoool of Medicine. Fishman played a directive role in all this work. Further discoveries culminated in his creation of the La Jolla Cancer Research Foundation in 1976. Fishman had decided to leave Tufts in order to strike out on his own. Starting from nothing in La Jolla and working almost with their bare hands, the Fishmans built what ultimately became one of the truly outstanding independent cancer research laboratories in the world.

That culminating achievement, against all odds, dismissed as impossible by Fishman's colleagues, is roughly where this story ends. It is also proof of the ultimate transformation of cancer research. In the years after World War I, biochemistry was seen as barely a step above animal husbandry, and yet it evolved into a vital tool of molecular biology permitting scientists to decode life-processes. All this occurred in the professional lifetime of one man. Moreover, the transformation reflected much of the substance of his own work.

What should we learn from these extraordinary changes?

• Fishman came from a family of deeply religious immigrant Jews. They brought with them all the sterling qualities of the Diaspora: commitment to hard work; love of family; a belief in education as the way to escape ignorance and poverty; reverence for their religion and culture. We must never cease revitalizing our nation by encouraging such people to settle here.

Throughout his lifetime Fishman struggled to build something that would remain after he was gone. This is the motivating ideal of every real scientist. It provides the strength to endure failure and disappointment. Wherever circumstances were unfavorable, Fishman persisted until eventually he achieved his dream of an independent laboratory. Now as university medical centers experience problems with financing research, and as the government slowly withdraws, Fishman's way seems to offer an approach in which American science can go on despite declining government support.

• Fishman was a dedicated scientist but he was no pushover, as his candid assessments of colleagues show. He battled for his ideas in New England and never found a completely friendly reception. He then took tremendous risks building a new laboratory in California. It demanded almost total commitment from Fishman and his wife, but somehow they succeeded. Others conspired to take his brainchild away from him. He fought them off. This breadth of competence is now rare as the scientific enterprise becomes narrowly specialized. We must continue to develop broad-guaged scientists capable of building not only models of nature, but laboratories. Specialization is important. Yet future leaders must know how to do more than science. Fishman had to solve every problem he encountered. Most of them were administrative things he never learned in school.

• When Fishman judged the right time had come in 1989, he retired, turning authority over to his successors. It is never easy to give up an enterprise you have built. The trustees of the La Jolla Cancer Research Foundation would gladly have welcomed him to stay on as President until the day he died. But Fishman understood that personal power is of little importance beside the best interests of an enduring institution. Knowing how and when to leave is a great leadership art, and it is also the mark of a great human being.

The La Jolla Cancer Research Foundation continues to thrive and grow on Torrey Pines Mesa. It is a unique creative achievement, centered on man's scientific struggle to overcome a deadly disease. It is also an organic monument to the energy, dedication, and wisdom of its founders.

Foreword by Sidney Weinhouse,
Professor Emeritus, Jefferson University, President 1981-2,
American Association for Cancer Research

The adage "Life begins at forty" has a parallel in the creation and remarkable success of the La Jolla Cancer Research Foundation, an inspiring saga of the fulfillment of William H. Fishman's dream, recounted in this volume.

When many men, even scientists are contemplating retirement, Bill Fishman, at 62, after 28 years as a research professor at Tufts Medical College, undertook a daunting challenge; the creation of a center of research to focus on a conception of cancer development which grew out of a lifetime of his research on the isoforms of alkaline phosphatase in experimental and human tumors.

He proposed that the bizarre growth of the neoplastic cells results from a defect in the precise orchestration of genetic expression occurring in normal embryonic development. Fetal protein expression in cancer was observed by others in various tumors, but received general acceptance only after the revolution in molecular genetics of the 80's and 90's.

Bill Fishman, convinced that rapid, further progress would require a degree of enthusiastic and concerted focus incompatible with the academic environment at Tufts, decided to create an independent organization. Resolved to set up shop in a center of excellence, he had the temerity to invade La Jolla, where such centers as the University of California at San Diego, The Salk Institute and the Scripps Institute were already flourishing. By a rare combination of hard work, dedication, ingenuity, an uncanny ability to recruit a stellar staff, and with the aid of Lillian Fishman, a biochemist in her own right and his wife and partner of 56 years, he was able to obtain generous community support; and taking advantage of timely deals on commercial property, the pygmy of La Jolla was transformed to a size and position of world respect.

In the meantime, the superb quality of science drew an incredible amount of peer-reviewed support from the NIH. A most opportune appointment was Erkki Ruoslahti, a world class scientist, who has taken over the reins as the second president of the Foundation after Bill's retirement in 1989. Bill credits him with "Building the scientific programs to their present prominence...".

Since its inception in 1976, it is recognized by the NCI as a basic cancer research center, has an annual budget of about $20 million, a staff of over a hundred scientists at the Ph.D. or M.D. level, and over a 3-year period, 1988-1991, it was third in the world in citations to their publications in the biomedical literature.

An engaging feature of this book is the history of the earlier Fishman family, a familiar story to many scientists of the Western world. Coming from Eastern Europe about 100 years ago, to escape the many hardships accompanied by frequent bloody pogroms, large elements of the Jewish population escaped to the West. The Fishman family, led by Bill's grandfather, settled in Manitoba, Canada, where the family eked out a marginal existence, but ultimately grew and prospered serving the mercantile needs of the wheat farmers of the region. In this respect they exhibited the very same qualities that characterized Bill's migration to La Jolla. Though money was scarce, love was abundant, Jewish religious principles were followed, education was permanent and hard work was necessary and expected.

In the rapidly expanding field of medical science today, the spotlight keeps moving from discovery to discovery of either potential or real benefit to the patient. What is not clearly recognized is the human struggle which precedes these reports or the characteristics of the research environment which are most important in nourishing the investigative efforts. This book is a fascinating account of one investigator's unique life journey which led to discoveries which formed the basis of founding one of the world's premier bioresearch institutions.

LIST OF PHOTOGRAPHS

INTRODUCTION

The Torrey Pine is one of the world's rarest trees. There are less than 6000 throughout the world. About 4000 of them are in the Torrey Pines State Reserve in La Jolla and in the reserve extension in Del Mar, California. The balance are on Santa Rosa island, 175 miles to the north of La Jolla.

Dr. C. C. Parry, a botanist, discovered the Torrey Pine in 1850. He named it Pinus Torreyana in honor of his friend and teacher, Dr. John Torrey of Columbia University.

Torrey Pines Mesa is located in the coastal strip of La Jolla in San Diego County.

If you were to stand in front of 10901 North Torrey Pines Road (La Jolla), in 1994, you would see five buildings hidden partially by a beautiful grove of Torrey pines on a nine acre plot of land. The entrance driveway is fronted by a sign "La Jolla Cancer Research Foundation.

These buildings are the workplace of some 300 employees, one hundred of whom are scientists with advanced degrees of Ph.D. or M.D. They come not only from the U.S.A., but from countries in Asia (Japan, China, Taiwan, India, Pakistan), Europe (Finland, Spain, Sweden, Germany, France, Switzerland, Russia, Poland), and the Middle East (Morocco, Egypt, Israel). Some 130,000 square feet of space houses the laboratories, offices and a library.

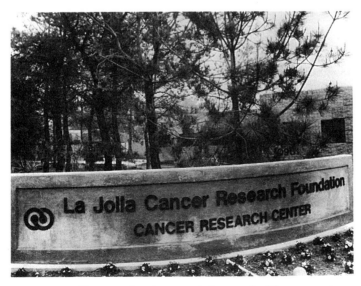

Monument sign at entrance to the grounds of the
La Jolla Cancer Research Foundation

The staff is composed of twenty-eight staff scientists, each of whom operates a laboratory supported by research grants from the National Institutes of Health, won in competition with their peers across the United States. The President and Chief Executive Officer is an internationally recognized scientist and administrator. The annual budget is in the realm of $20,000,000 and three of the five buildings were built since 1985 to accommodate the growing successful research program.

The Board of Trustees number twenty-five community leaders drawn from business, the professions, and the philanthropists of San Diego and Los Angeles.

The Foundation, established in 1976, has been operating since 1981 its National Cancer Institute Basic Science Cancer Research Center; of which there are only fourteen in the whole United States. In a recent ranking of institutions by the Citation Index (an objective measure of the attention given by scientists to the value of research publications) for the ten year period 1981-1991, La Jolla Cancer Research Foundation was seventh. For the more recent three- year period (1988-91), the Foundation ranked third in the world. The rapidity with which an Institution achieved this recognition on practically no start-up funds is unprecedented.

It should be remembered that in the year La Jolla Cancer Research Foundation was founded there existed three flourishing research institutions in La Jolla which were in the process of establishing their own cancer centers. The University of California at San Diego had a star-studded Faculty and Dr. John Mendelsohn, was the first Director of its clinical center. The Salk Institute which has the most Nobel Prize winners of any Institution of comparable size, operated the Armand Hammer Cancer Center headed by Dr. Walter Eckhardt. At the prestigious Scripps Clinic and Research Foundation, a basic science cancer center had been organized by Dr. Frank Huennekens. (Today, this institution has become the world's largest private institution devoted to basic research in disease.)

How did the La Jolla Cancer Research Foundation manage to succeed in this environment, let alone survive? Trustee, William Drell has stated, "It was a miracle."

At this point, I wish to share with the reader a few relevant thoughts.

Some years ago I came across a statement printed on parchment paper which was sold in drug stores and stationery shops. To me it was an arresting statement. The more I thought about it, the more I found myself identifying with it. It reads

PRESS ON

"Nothing in this world can take the place of persistence. Talent will not; nothing is more common than unsuccessful men with talent. Genius will not; unrewarded genius is almost a proverb. Education will not; the world is full of educated derelicts. Persistence and determination alone are omnipotent. The slogan "press on" has solved and always will solve the problems of the human race."

CALVIN COOLIDGE

In recent years a number of people who heard the story of the creation of the La Jolla Cancer Research Foundation have urged me to describe it in a book. As I reflect on the philosophical basis of the founding of this institution, I kept recalling the theme of the "Press On" statement. It seemed to me that readers would be better able to understand where the Foundation came from if they had knowledge of the history of the people who were its founders and the role of the "Press On" theme. This book is an attempt to tell the story.

Cancer researchers had not always been highly regarded in the scientific community in mid-century as they are now. At that time, such individuals were regarded as second-class scientists. Why does one choose to become a cancer researcher when one is already recognized as a first class promising scientist? This is the story of one such individual.

"Only in America" is a phrase which is often repeated by many of us who have identified opportunities and were able to achieve success way beyond our dreams. It was the creation of the National Institutes of Health; and the introduction of the peer review system which offered research opportunity to scientists who merited it regardless of academic politics, cronyism, race, religion, or country of origin. We all owe a debt to the far-sighted legislators who passed the law creating the National Institutes of Health. The challenge of writing NIH grant applications in competition with scientists all over the country, the pleasure in receiving a fundable priority score on peer review and the opportunity to perform research towards achieving stated specific aims animate all of us and fosters independent thinking. This process is repeated many times during a scientific career. What happens when a grant is not funded? What resources can the scientist marshall in the interim? Can a scientist at age sixty-two compete with one age thirty-two, in the arena of new testable ideas? This is the story of such a survivor who did.

In the market place of ideas, I have been a witness to the statement that nothing is as powerful as an idea whose time has come. This is to a large extent the secret of the creation of the La Jolla Cancer Research Foundation. It has been pointed out to me that it was a scientific concept, "the oncodevelopmental concept," which produced this institution and which distinguishes it from its counterparts in universities, medical schools, and hospitals. Many have told me, "Fishman, you have been the right person, with the right idea, at the right place and at the right time."

Several years ago, I watched on the TV screen a documentary on navigation. Pictured was a modern-day naval frigate with a missile launcher armed and ready to be fired. It was moving in a circle, back and forth. In the command cabin, a navigator was poring over a map. Said the commentator, "We can't fix the course and destination of this missile unless we know exactly where we are." "Where we are" needed to be defined in terms of the coordinates of latitude and longitude on a map.

It struck me forcibly later that in one's journey through life, one cannot attempt to reach a distant goal unless one objectively identifies where one is presently located in this path of life. Once this has been defined, one can examine two questions. How did we get here? and How do we now get from here to the distant goal? These are the questions which will be examined here. Each chapter will define a milestone or "navigational fix" followed by a recollection of how it was reached. This book is essentially an autobiographical story which is justified only to the extent that it helps the reader understand the genesis of the La Jolla Cancer Research Foundation.

In 1937, I met in western Canada the one who eventually became the co-founder of the La Jolla Cancer Research Foundation. Lillian Waterman is a beautiful, enthusiastic and charming woman with a strong interest in science.

Another unique personal note is that our marriage is intact and thriving after fifty-six years, a measure of our mutual devotion and commitment. Thus, from 1939 on, my wife, Lillian, shared in every way the triumphs, disappointments, hardships, anxieties, and unremitting effort. She is an individual of great integrity, strong determination, warm personality, and complete devotion to our personal and professional goals.

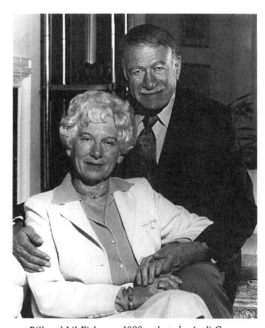

Bill and Lil Fishman, 1989 - photo by A. di Gesu

Basically this book relates the "Bill and Lil Story" and the events leading to and following the creation of the La Jolla Cancer Research Foundation. As we enter our eighth decade, we have asked ourselves, "If not now, when?" That is why this book is written now!

It is also necessary to place this story in the context of the ever-changing picture of science in America over the past sixty years with its current explosion of new information of the nature of genes and the control of their expression. In a sense the "Bill and Lil" story is a case history of their path over this interval through the labyrinthine structure of society, government, academia and industry. At every turn of the way, there were set-backs which were overcome only by a greater devotion to the challenge of the research and to our personal integrity. Perhaps there is a lesson here for the young scientist at the beginning of a career who may find the traditional steps of advancement intimidating and too restrictive to one's research opportunity. Related also are the rewards and costs of embarking on a research project which is far from the popular fields of research led by the power structure elite. In time, if the publications appear in first-class journals in sufficient numbers, recognition eventually comes and with it the ability to compete for peer-reviewed NIH grants on merit only.

In short, the concept, the commitment to discovery, the enhancement of the research opportunity for each member of the staff remains the motivating principles of the institution and its leadership. Dr. Erkki Ruoslahti, currently the President and Chief Executive Officer is carrying forward this commitment in a most imaginative and creative manner.

I have on occasion wondered if this volume deserves a place in the company of Nobel Prize winners who have written their autobiographies and have described how they had cleverly wrested important secrets from the grasp of nature. However, I have been comforted by a remark to me by Dr. Ruoslahti. It was after a meeting of our Board of Scientific Advisors which included a Nobel Prize winner and several members of the Nobel Prize class. I expressed my admiration and respect for these towering figures of science. Ruoslahti told me very firmly—"there isn't one of the lot who could have done what you have accomplished with LJCRF".

This then is not an account of the rarified intellectual competitive environment of the ivory tower and the winners in that climate. It is rather a view of the "outsider" who had a commitment to a scientific mission and together with his spouse created a home, different from any other, in which this mission could be pursued successfully. We believe that when the final chapter on the conquest of cancer is written, this Foundation will be credited with having made a major contribution.

As to the organization of this book, it divides itself into two parts. The first (Chapters 1 through 11) reviews in chronological order the events which formed my perspective on scientific research and which led to my appointment to a research professorship at Tufts University in 1948 at age 35. Included also are my efforts over 28 years culminating in the creation of the Tufts Cancer Research Center. Finally, the second part (Chapters 12-20) describes the founding of the La Jolla Cancer Research Foundation in which there has been a coalescence of scientific oncologic concepts, a unique organizational structure and a dynamic leadership. This leadership has since 1989 been in the hands of Dr. Erkki Ruoslahti, the second President of LJCRF, and who merits the credit of building the scientific programs to their present prominence and who pioneered in the fields of adhesive proteins and integrins, a major subject of widespread interest today.

PART I

THE FOUNDERS

CHAPTER 1

MY ROOTS, ABE AND GOLDIE, WINNIPEG, OAKBURN

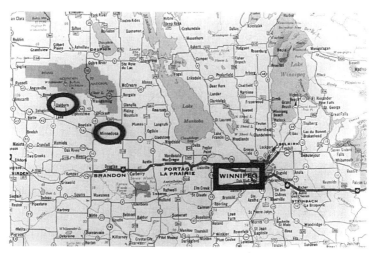

Location of Winnipeg, Minnedosa and Oakburn in the province of Manitoba, Canada
(Map ©1980 by Rand McNally, R.L. 95-S-270.)

It was a bitterly cold winter day in Winnipeg on March 2, 1914 when Goldie Fishman brought me into the world. This is our first milestone date fixed by the coordinates of time, geography and parents.

Who was Abe Fishman? Who was Goldie Chmelnitsky, his bride, and where did they come from? Their roots are my roots.

The first Abraham Fishman, born in 1760, was descended from the Spanish Jews fleeing the Spanish Inquisition of 1492, lived in Ladyzen, Russia. His son, Hershvelv (1830-1887) was a miller of buckwheat—Yitschak Joel (1852-1927), his grandson, lived in Petosk where he married Sara Doba Segal in 1880. They operated an inn and then moved to Poniatovka, some 30 miles from Odessa. Sara's grandfather came from Lithuania where he was the head teacher of the Vilna Yeshiva. Yitschak Joel Fishman and his family reached Winnipeg in 1908, fugitives from the Russian pogroms. They spent the first years operating a dairy farm in Kildonan several miles north of Winnipeg.

The family was very observant in their religious practices. The extent of this statement can be judged by this recollection. Observant Jews did not ride on the Sabbath yet milk had to be delivered to households in Winnipeg every day. Abe Fishman at age 20 would walk beside the milk wagon the entire delivery route in the heat of summer and in the bitter cold of winter and instruct the driver where to deliver the milk on Saturdays.

The family then moved to Winnipeg which had a sizeable Jewish community and operated a grocery store.

On my mother's side, her earliest identifiable ancestor was an Abraham Chmelnitsky who lived from 1850-1901 in Novakrainka, Russia. He was a well-known cantor and his son, Israel Moses, my grandfather, became a lumber merchant. He was married to Rivka Podell. They arrived in Winnipeg in 1905 and operated a general store in Poplar Point. Their oldest, daughter, Goldie, fell in love with the young hardy handsome milkman, Abe Fishman, and they were married on January 12, 1912.

ABE AND GOLDIE

My recollections of my father and mother are dimmed by the many years which have elapsed since their deaths but certain highlights will never fade.

My father was a physically powerful man and a morally righteous person. He was highly literate in Russian and Ukrainian and was respected and liked by the farmers in Oakburn who had immigrated from the "old country." His years in Oakburn (1912-1925) traversed World War I, the ravaging Spanish

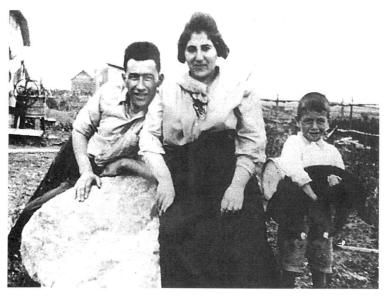

Abe and Goldie Fishman with Bill holding a dog - Oakburn circa 1920

influenza epidemic and the rapid growth of wheat farming in Manitoba. He told of the demands of the bank for immediate payment of a major loan and how he liquidated the lumberyard and other assets in three days to pay off the bank. His good name and its preservation had the highest priority.

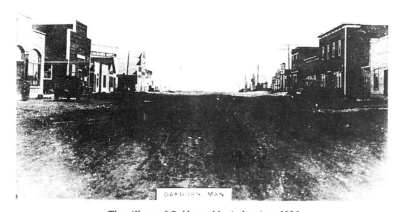

The village of Oakburn, Manitoba circa 1920

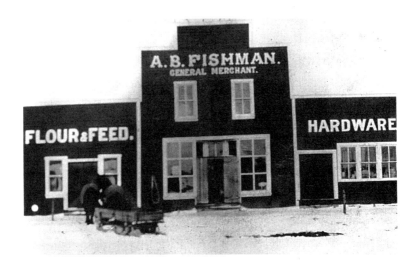

To generate income outside of the general store, he would accept butter and eggs from farmers in exchange for merchandise. Each Sunday morning he processed the week's collection of butter by the washing techniques he knew as a dairyman and shipped a top grade barrel of butter to the Winnipeg market. Cattle hides, furs, and Seneca roots were also bartered for goods.

The age of the automobile arrived and brought with it scenes of cars stuck in Manitoba mud roads. A team of horses would be recruited from a nearby farm to attempt to retrieve autos from the ditch alongside the road. The story is told of the inability of the horses to pull our neighbor's car out of the ditch. Abe positioned himself with his back to the rear bumper, grasped it with both hands and lifted the rear of the vehicle to the point that the horses were able to pull the car back on the road.

He did not tolerate insults to his Jewish heritage or his religion and has been reported to have thrown his disparagers bodily out of the store - after which no one dared to denigrate him.

Goldie Fishman was a warm-hearted, hospitable woman who devoted herself completely to Abe and the children. Saul was the oldest, I followed one year later and Isobel, sixteen years later.

Mother was an able diplomat, she succeeded in calming tempers of individual members of the family and maintained the peace. She possessed a fine soprano voice and both she and Abe would sing the popular tunes of the day, most regularly during outings in the car.

Two major guidelines were taught us. One was to respect and to observe the "Ten Commandments" of the Bible and the other admonition was "Where there is a will, there is a way!" My parents set an example for us of consideration for other people's views and of the joy of independence.

In business Abe counted seventeen partners in various enterprises in which his role varied from grain broker, horse trader, lumberman, farmer, dairyman, and merchant. With one exception all of the partners were either relatives or close friends. The exception was a Scotsman, A. G. Clark, with whom Abe shared ownership of "the Cash store" in Minnedosa, Manitoba. They got along beautifully and Abe was admitted to the Masonic Lodge, Goldie to the Eastern Star organization; both played badminton, golf, and bridge. They were very well liked.

Family was very important to Abe and Goldie. Goldie had a sister, Bessie, Abe, a sister, Bonnie, both in Saskatoon. This circumstance was a major factor motivating the family's move to Saskatoon. Another factor was the availability of the University of Saskatchewan in the same city for Saul and I to attend. Abe and Goldie did everything in their power to provide their children with a good education. Their deep regret was that they themselves did not receive a formal education-yet they taught themselves to read and to write fluently in English.

WINNIPEG

Winnipeg at that time was the gateway to Western Canada. The Canadian Pacific Railroad transported thousands of immigrants from the port city of Montreal to Western Canada. For many it was an opportunity to own and farm land under the Homestead Act. A settler could own 160 acres of land if over a period of three years, he cleared a number of acres and planted them with grain crops.

According to Pierre Berton's "The Promised Land" (1), Winnipeg by 1911 was at the peak of a railroad boom with two dozen tracks leading out from the city. There were not enough railroad cars to carry all the wheat which poured in from the prairie provinces, even with 15,500 freight cars. The population was imbued with a spirit of enthusiastic optimism and a land and building boom resulted from the railroad's support of the economy.

The spirit of the West was defined as enthusiasm, optimism and energy balanced with a healthy sincerity. The focus of attention for all was the status of the "Crop" which included wheat, barley and oats. Even when the crops of whole districts were repeatedly wiped out by heavy spring rain, rust fungus and hail- even when some crops had survived, all were at risk of an early frost, Western farmers shrugged their shoulders and said "next year we will have a bumper crop!" This attitude was pervasive during the first half of the 20th century.

Aside from Winnipeg being a hub of two railroads; the Canadian Pacific Railway and the Canadian National Railway; it was located also at the junction of two rivers. From the western plains there was the Assinaboine river and from North Dakota, the Red river flowed. They joined together to empty into Lake Winnipeg. In the early days, Fort Gary, a Royal Mounted Police headquarters and trading post was the destination of Indians and trappers from all directions.

In the city itself, two main traffic arteries met in the heart of the city - one was Main street servicing the northern part of the city and the other was Portage Avenue which led to Brandon and points West. Both were exceptionally wide streets, a tribute to the foresight of the early city planners.

It was understandable that many immigrants chose to make Winnipeg their home. It was the first opportunity to escape from the crowded colonist coaches in which they were trapped for four days and four nights on the transcontinental trips from Montreal. At the end of each coach was an iron stove and a coal bin. This device which generated more smoke than fire was the source of heat, and a place to attempt to cook food.

OAKBURN

The big event of the day was the arrival of the train from Winnipeg. It came three times a week to Oakburn, a village of 50 souls. This is where Abe Fishman took his wife in 1912 and established A.B. Fishman's General Store.

About 30 minutes before the train's arrival, one began to notice movements of people and wagons, much as the concentric travels of iron filings towards a magnet. A crowd assembled on the station platform. Inside the station one could hear the clickity-clak-clik-clik of the telegraph key as it spoke in its staccato voice to the telegraph operator and as he replied in kind. What mysterious messages were being transmitted?

The baggage master wheeled out a huge wagon onto the station platform and drew it to a location where he expected the baggage car to stop. On his cart there was a variety of items; cream cans, boxes of henna root, piles of cow hides, and passenger valises and trunks.

"There she is!" cried one of the spectators. Down the straight stretch of track one could glimpse a tiny cloud of smoke. To our ears drifted the faint sounds of the whistle being blown at each road crossing... whooo-whooo-who-whoooo.

As the train neared the station we were threatened by a continuously clanging bell and the escape of white steam from each side of the engine, rapidly engulfing the viewers. Cinders fell on us all. The passengers who dismounted the passenger coach, were met by their families, collected their baggage and departed. The baggageman then transferred his load to the train, and in turn, unloaded things like machinery parts, boxes of harness items, animal traps and boxes of canned goods for the general store.

With the cry of "All Aboard" from the conductor the train shuddered as the fly-wheel of the locomotive struggled to create a forward movement. Slowly, slowly the train moved out to the accompaniment of a series of "choo-choo's" heard in an ever increasing frequency. It began to recede in the distance on its way to Rossburn, the next set of grain elevators to the West. The telegraph key in the station continued to click-clack in its conversation with operators up and down the railroad line in the midst of tranquil silence.

Life in Oakburn was pleasant for Saul and I. Sunday was the day for the family. Lunch was the big event. Often, Goldie would serve a delicious pot roast which produced a tasty gravy. It was separated, fortified with garlic and poured hot over freshly baked rolls which were named "pompishkes". At other times the gravy enriched the "veranekes" whose closest relatives are the "Wonton" of the Chinese cuisine. After dinner, all of us went for a two mile walk and enjoyed the fresh air.

At other times, Sunday was the time to visit and be visited. In Elphinstone, a two hour drive from Oakburn lived Abe's youngest sister, Bonnie—married to Morris Lerman. Also in Shoal Lake lived the Zivot family. Both Lermans and Zivot's operated small general stores. At each visit, a magnificent feast was shared and much conversation and jokes.

We acquired a Victrola which when cranked up adequately would produce wonderful music from thick record platters. Goldie cherished the operas especially those starring Enrico Caruso and also light operas like "die Fledermaus".

Abe built our home in Oakburn with two new features at the time. The home was powered by a stack of batteries and it had indoor plumbing leading to an underground cesspool, located many feet underground below the frost line.

I have many good memories of our family experiences in Oakburn.

CHAPTER 2

LIFE ON THE PRAIRIES IN THE '30s

There definitely were four seasons on the prairies, each with its own unmistakable character.

Winter in the country was somewhat different from winter in the city. As one looked out of the frost encrusted windows in Oakburn one could see the wind-whipped waves of snow, resembling the white-capped waves of the sea stirred by gale force winds. When the wind died down, one could walk on the hard surface of the three foot snow drifts without falling through. The children attending the one-room school house one mile south of town, made igloos by fashioning snow blocks from the snow banks. The horse-drawn sleigh was the school bus in those days. More pleasant were the horse-drawn enclosed sleds with foot warmers and blankets which traversed the roads accompanied by the sound of tinkling sleigh bells.

In the city, the snow-filled streets and side walks were navigated by sleds. Very rarely was school cancelled because of blizzard conditions. Transportation by street car was affordable by few...and automobile travel was precarious at best since the streets were not plowed. Woolen underwear, socks, pants, and sweaters separated one's body from the heavy overcoat, scarf with a woolen toque covering the head. Indian moccasins were the desired footwear. Travel to school was by foot only.

March 21, the first official day of spring, witnessed considerable amounts of snow still on the ground but as the days grew longer and the sun rose higher in the sky there was some melting. The water immediately froze when the night temperature fell to below zero degrees Fahrenheit. Thus, in the morning, one found little ponds of clear hard ice between the snow banks. By

April, the challenge to the pedestrian was how to navigate between ever wider and deeper pools of ice water and still use the sidewalk. Many times, children and even adults slipped and fell into the icy water.

May 24, Queen Victoria's birthday, was notable because by then the frost had left the ground and both farmers and home gardeners prepared the soil for the first planting. Plowing could be seriously delayed because of heavy spring rains which would fill the sloughs and low regions of the land. These provided the habitat for ducks and geese migrating from the south. The arrival of robins, meadow larks and other avian song species produced a quickening of the heartbeat in many a gardener and farmer. This was also the season for seeing the mares with their attached suckling colts, the cows with their newborn ungainly calves, and hens and ducks with their many progeny following the mother bird Indian file everywhere she went.

The measure of summer was the height of the stand of wheat, oats, and barley at any particular time. By the first of July, a good crop was at least two feet high and was beginning to "head out" *i.e.* to form the grain kernels in the mass of protruding whiskers of these plants. By mid-August, the crop was ripe for "binding and stooking." The binder, pulled by a team of horses, cut the wheat about six inches from the ground and secured the sheaves with twine. These were deposited in rows behind the binder and the farm hands would stand up the sheaves in a type of pyramid or "stook."

The exciting time was the harvest when a steam engine would power the threshing machine with its huge belts. The ripe sheaves were forked into this machine. A wagon fitted with wooden sides, three feet high, received the streams of golden grain. There were many men in the threshing crews and they often worked well into the night to take advantage of the good weather and also to be in a position to service the next farm. Trainloads of workers would travel from Eastern Canada to man the collection of the harvest. They were housed and fed by the farmers. As the grain wagons were filled, they were horse driven to the grain elevators. The farmer received a receipt for the number of bushels delivered and this could be exchanged for a check based on the market price for wheat, oats, or barley that day. Such pay days were followed by the settling up of accumulated debts at the country store, blacksmith, farm, physician, machinery company, etc.

Money was scarce! What counted was "a good name." With a good name, the wholesale distributors would extend credit to buy merchandise, allowing a merchant to stay in business so long as he paid his bills. This applied to everyone.

How did the family retain its Jewish identity and heritage? Saul and I were boarded with Abe's parents in Winnipeg for a few years so that we could attend Hebrew school for two hours a day during the week and religious services on the Sabbath. Eventually, the Fishman family sold the business in Oakburn and moved to Winnipeg. It was during this Winnipeg interval to 1927 that we reinforced our family relationships especially with Abe's married sisters, Dinah (Levin) and Baila (Lucow) and their families. We literally had cousins by the dozen with whom we played and socialized. Harry, my cousin, and Myrna Levin have remained our closest friends over the years.

The following events made 1927 memorable: I became Bar Mitzvah at age 13, my grandfather, Yitschak Joel Fishman died, and we moved to Minnedosa where Abe returned to being a merchant.

MINNEDOSA

Minnedosa was regarded as a major town in Western Manitoba. It was a division point of the Canadian Pacific Railroad and at least two trains a day in each direction stopped at the depot in the center of town. One mile away was the reservoir and a dam with a power station, at the outlet of which one could usually catch a couple of jackfish. Fishing tackle was crude—a bamboo pole with 6 feet of fishing line ending with a hook and a lead sinker attached at the very end of the line. Bait was usually a sliver of bacon fat, or a live worm or small frog. Fishing was my hobby.

We often played golf on a nine hole course—with bamboo shafted clubs and on "greens" which were oiled sand expanses that one was required to smooth over after "holing out" so that those following would have an unspoiled "green" for putting. Saul excelled in the game and developed a life-time habit of shooting in the low 80's.

The Minnedosa Collegiate Institute was the name of the high school. It was staffed by an elite group of no-nonsense mature teachers who demanded our best efforts. My brother Saul is blessed with a very fine intellect and he was advanced by two grades in one year. He won the Governor General's medal which was given to the one who achieved by graduation, the most in scholarship, sports and general all-around citizenship.

Two years later, I found that Saul was a hard act to follow. To master my subjects in High School, I had to work three times as hard. Although I was by no means an athlete, there were two areas in which I could compete: one was the one mile race and the other was ice hockey.

To prepare myself for the one-mile race, I would trot out to the fair-grounds, circle the track for the one mile distance and trot back home for breakfast. On the day of the high school's track competition, I was confident but had made the mistake of wearing a jock-strap for the very first time. A field of ten took off with the starter's gun. The day was sunny but a 20 mile-an-hour wind was blowing in from the west. With the handicap of the annoying jock-strap and the wind, I fell steadily behind the leading runner. The first and second place racers had already crossed the finish line and I was still 100 yards out, laboring mightily. I just managed to finish the race when I collapsed. No other participants crossed the finish line. Perhaps, others would point to this episode as evidence that "Bill is a plugger"; my Dad did.

In high school hockey, the poorest skater ended up as the goalie, protecting the net. I was really under-qualified for this position but was reasonably successful. My undoing came when the men's hockey team took the ice after our high school game and recruited me to defend one goal net. The pads which I wore provided no protection from the high-velocity missile (the puck) which the men fired at me. I survived the ordeal but with some severe bruises.

When I graduated in 1931, it was a triumph to learn that like my brother, I had won the Governor-General's medal and an Isbister Scholarship to defray the tuition for the freshman year at the University of Manitoba. However, as fate decreed, I spent my freshman year at the University of Saskatchewan when the family moved to Saskatoon.

Minnedosa was a milestone for another reason. In 1930, on November 8, my sister Isobel was born. I was 16 years older than my sister with whom I formed a life-long bond. Saul was away at the University of Manitoba during Isobel's first year and I was a resource to mother.

CHAPTER 3

THE UNIVERSITY OF SASKATCHEWAN (1931-1935)

Situated east of the broad Saskatchewan river and the metropolis of Saskatoon, numbering some 40,000 inhabitants, was a cluster of new buildings of limestone constructed in Gothic style. This was the University of Saskatchewan. It was only 20 years old.

It was there that I took my first course, General Chemistry, taught by a Professor A. C. Fraser whose enthusiasm and ability to make chemistry a live subject, coupled with laboratory exercises, attracted my serious attention. The order of the elements in Mendeleev's table, the laws of mass action and conservation of matter, Avogadro's number, kinetic theory of chemical reactions, all aroused in me wonder and appreciation of the order of the world we live in. Each chemistry course, qualitative and quantitative analysis, physical and colloid chemistry, organic and biochemistry added building blocks of knowledge which opened up a new world for me. I found biochemistry most interesting as it encompassed the chemistry of life. It was Dr. Roger Manning who described in his biochemistry course such vivid examples as fermentation, and insulin action; studies which preceded our awareness of intermediary metabolism.

I was very impressed with the intellect and character of a student who also graduated with high honors in chemistry in 1935. He was able to grasp new concepts in chemistry many times faster than I. This required me to work that much harder to keep up with him. As the academic year was drawing to a close in April, my colleague told me how much he looked forward to planting the wheat on his parents' farm. This fellow was Henry Taube (2) who later won the Nobel Prize in Chemistry. He is now Professor Emeritus of Chemistry at Stanford University.

A number of us lived about three miles from the University. In the midst of below-zero winter weather you could see us striding rapidly to the 25th Avenue bridge and braving the last mile over the wind-swept prairie before reaching the shelter of the University buildings. No one ever took the street car even though the fare was 5¢. Why? Nobody had 5¢ to spare.

Upon graduation in 1935, I was determined to do biochemical research. Just how this step was implemented is now described.

In 1935, my father moved the family from Saskatoon to Oakburn, Manitoba, where we lived on the south half of section 2 North. The farm consisted of a two-story frame house, a barn, and a well with its windmill. The depression on the prairies was widespread and my father had liquidated his business in Saskatoon, paying all his creditors. The move to the farm reduced the cost of living significantly and it also made it possible for him to manage his considerable land possessions—at one time amounting to 17 quarter sections of land. Meanwhile, my brother Saul had finished law school at the University of Saskatchewan and moved to Moose Jaw to article in a lawyer's office, at zero salary. Many starving lawyers in those days went into other lines of work to make a living.

My father was alert to the opportunities of scientific agriculture. He especially was interested in animal husbandry; upgrading the stocks of cattle, as well as developing better breeds of horses and sheep. His desire was for me to enter into partnership in providing a breeding service to the farmers in Oakburn and environs.

He also was anxious to have his children become as educated as possible. Evidence for this was his purchase in the 1920's of leather-bound sets of the complete works of William Shakespeare,

Rudyard Kipling and the many volumes of the Harvard Classics.

In the summer of 1935 after graduation, I worked as a farm hand, "stooking" the wheat sheaves, growing a vegetable garden, etc.

One evening my father and I were perched on the rail fence of the farm. It was twilight. Dad had a paid-up life insurance policy of $750 which he offered to me to use in whatever way I decided was best; either to join in the animal husbandry enterprise or to pursue graduate education. I responded that I wanted to see if I had any ability to do biochemical research. This could be ascertained in one year of graduate study. If I lacked this ability I would return to the farm and happily become a partner with Dad. And so we reached another milestone.

CHAPTER 4

BIOCHEMISTRY IN TORONTO

GETTING THERE

Uncle Louis, my father's older brother, drove me in his pick-up truck from Oakburn to the Winnipeg stockyards. He was a cattle trader which entitled him to send a representative to accompany his cattle from Winnipeg to the Toronto market. I was lucky to be that person. We traveled all night.

The huge harvest moon in September lit up the grain fields which now were populated by numerous small pyramids of wheat sheaves. In the distance one could see the busy threshing machines around which were clustered men, horses and wagons illuminated by burning mounds of straw. This trip from Oakburn to Winnipeg was the first step in my journey into the exploration of life, science, and the world which lay beyond the prairies.

NEXT MORNING

Carrying my single suitcase, I found the train registration area in the Winnipeg stockyards. After a while I emerged with signed papers giving me permission to accompany 100 head of cattle to Toronto and to look after their welfare. That evening several of us boarded a caboose which was then shunted back and forth till it reached its destination at the back end of a long line of Canadian Pacific Railway freight cars including the cattle cars.

A motley group of men representing other cattle traders were my companions on that journey. Several appeared to me to be men about town of the sporting type. Their language was explosive and punctuated by obscenities. If one believed their exploits, they posed as characters before whom women swooned immediately with passion and surrendered. Others were inveterate gamblers and their poker game proceeded with few interruptions through the whole journey.

The colonist cars were fitted with seats and backs which could be arranged horizontally into makeshift beds. The windows did not fit very well and the passengers were often the targets of streams of cinders cascading in from the steam locomotives. By morning, the car was very cold especially when the train passed through northern Ontario. We took turns keeping the coal fire burning in the iron stove at the end of the coach.

There was no food service of any kind on this cattle train. A half-day stop at White River Junction, Ontario, provided an opportunity to buy food and supplies for the rest of the journey. We were all happy to arrive in Toronto— tired, hungry, dirty, and unshaven.

A COOL RECEPTION AT THE
UNIVERSITY OF TORONTO

To my knowledge, I had completed the registration forms to enter the graduate school and had mailed them two months before the start of the fall semester. However, although I had received no reply, I decided to go to Toronto and, if not accepted, to apply to other institutions.

My first priority then was to visit the Department of Biochemistry and to find out whether or not I had been accepted into its graduate program. I found myself stating this question to the secretary of the Department.

Miss Molly Delamere was a formidable character who demanded that I explain why I had not answered her letter. Since I had not received it, I suggested that because the train brought the mail to Oakburn three times a week, the letter might have arrived after I left. She refused to accept this suggestion repeating over and over again, "You did receive my letter! Why didn't you answer it?"

I then asked very politely if I could see Dr. Hardolph Wasteneys, the Chairman of the Department. Very reluctantly she ushered me into his impressive office.

Dr. Wasteneys was seated behind a massive desk and gruffly said, "Sit down, Fishman." He then looked at my scholastic records, growled for several seconds and then exclaimed, "Good marks aren't enough! I need letters of recommendation from your Saskatchewan professors. Until I receive them, you are not admitted to graduate school... but, in the meantime, you can audit the required courses. Good day, Fishman."

Two weeks later, Dr. Wasteneys informed me that I was qualified to do graduate studies in biochemistry. But how was I to find out if I could do research in order to determine whether or not to return to the farm in a year? The opportunity came in a course on enzymology (the study of enzymes) which Professor Arthur M. Wynne taught. There was the possibility of doing a laboratory thesis for a minor in enzymology.

Dr. Wynne had become expert in the fermentation of corn suspensions by the microorganism *clostridium acetobutylicum* which produced acetone and butyl alcohol in large quantities. This fermentation was the means by which the Allies in World War I were able to manufacture acetone, a major requirement in the process of making explosives. These original cultures were prepared by Dr. Chaim Weizmann who later became the first president of the State of Israel. The Balfour Declaration was in large part Britain's reward to Dr. Weizmann. It stated that His Majesty's Government viewed with favor the establishment of a home in Palestine for the Jewish people. Little did I or anybody imagine that the State of Israel would be created and would thrive as a consequence of this declaration and that I would be studying the activity of a microorganism with such historical significance.

The sampling of the fermentation at two-hour intervals proceeded for 36 hours or more. This was my introduction to all-night endeavors, a characteristic at that time of the requirements of many research projects. The results were sufficiently interesting to yield a thesis (3) which had merit. I knew then that my direction would be biochemistry and not animal husbandry.

Life in Toronto started off with a setback. I was crossing St. George Street when I was hit by a taxi which was going too fast. My head met the pavement with a thud. The resulting gash over my right eye required ten stitches to close. My landlady was very surprised to see me return with a bloody bandaged head. I am always careful in crossing streets now!

Imagine my naiveté on the ways of the real world when I accepted the terms of the taxicab company to settle my case—$19.95 for a new pair of pants to replace the ones torn in the crash.

In 1936, Canada was still in the depths of the great depression and I was worried as to how I might continue in graduate school once the $750 was spent. It was wonderful to learn that for the next year I would have an appointment as "demonstrator" in Biochemistry and would be teaching the medical students in the laboratory. Few graduate students won this opportunity. The stipends started at $600 and reached $800 per annum at my graduation. I was lucky to have this support for three years.

With these riches, I could afford to share a furnished apartment with another graduate student, Ben Schachter, travel yearly to Vancouver where the Fishman family then lived, for a one-month vacation, and to save some money.

CAMARADERIE

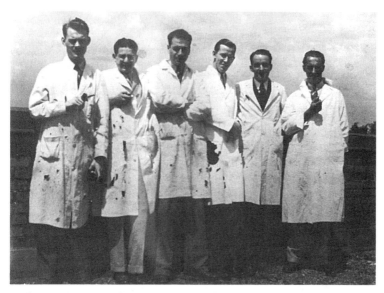

Graduate students in Biochemistry, University of Toronto, 1938 (l. to r.): Gord Butler, Benny Schachter, Bill Fishman, Art Odell, Marv Darrach, Professor Guy F. Marrian

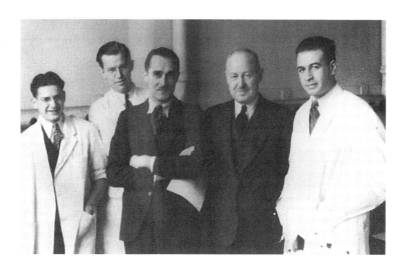

(l. to r.): Benny Schachter, Art Odell, Professor Guy F. Marrian, Professor A.M. Wynne and Bill Fishman - 1938

Everyone in and out of the research laboratory was friendly during those years... perhaps because we were all in the same boat... nobody had any money and so there was no envy.

Much of my social life was centered in two circles of friends. One was composed of my contemporaries from Saskatoon and the prairies who had entered the University of Toronto and the other was made up of my fellow graduate students.

My prairie friends would get together to participate in the Jewish High Holy Days, in the Passover Seder, and in other festivities, i.e., birthdays.

My colleagues in the department were an interesting crew with good communication and good-will being the rule. We begin with Dr. Wasteneys who in his earlier days had been a chemist inspector of tea in India. He once told us of his discovery that iron filings often were used to adulterate the tea. He later had held an appointment at the Rockefeller Institute. He was at his best presiding over the departmental tea which was served at 4 P.M. and attended by the entire staff. He was a highly principled kindhearted man who set the tone for the entire staff.

Dr. Wasteneys was active in the Department from 1918-1947 and created an environment in which scholarship could and did flourish. A measure of the stature of this man can be obtained from a statement he made at his Tribute Dinner on May 26, 1947.

> "Well, we tried to give you here the best we could of training in biochemistry and in biochemical research. That was our first and bounden duty. But for myself, I should feel more happy if I were always sure that we had contributed also to the development of your character; that we had helped you to achieve a sense of purpose in your lives, that we had taught you to feel that good workmanship and solid accomplishment were in themselves worthwhile ends, that you had learnt to value the approval of your peers in Science before the meretricious and evanescent

acclaim of the daily press. I should feel happy if I knew that we had helped you to achieve a sense of values which might guide you towards some contribution to a solution of the problems of our troubled world. Science is our vocation! true, and we must follow it. Nonetheless, the great need of our world today is not more science, but a marriage of science and humanism (and transcendentalism too, if you must have it) in a new and true religion, to the end that we may at last achieve a real "brotherhood of Man" and be freed from the "slough of despond" in which we now wallow. Oh! I know our Governments and our Governors, today are protesting that science, scientists, and our universities, for a while, they say, must sacrifice many of their ideals to the imminent needs of National Defense and National Industry. But what shall it profit us, if we gain the world to lose our souls. I pray too, that in this new era of highly organized, highly specialized, highly oriented research, our successors may not be discouraged from pursuing those exciting and glorious adventures of the mind and spirit which have made our lives so worth living. The danger that this may happen is not immediately apparent, but I think it is real."

Dr. Wasteneys exemplified the marriage of science and humanism and all of us were molded by his values. I was! His words were prophetic!

The star researcher of the Department was Professor Guy F. Marrian from London. He was a tall, tanned, lithe, athletic man with a pair of green eyes which shone like headlights when he spoke to you. He was a co-discoverer of estrogenic steroids and together with E. A. Doisy of St. Louis and A. Butenandt of

Germany proved the four-ring structure of the steroid hormones. He attracted a large number of bright, highly-motivated graduate students who advanced knowledge in the estrogenic steroids in relation to pregnancy. From the first students, Saul L. Cohen and Desmond Beall, there followed Gordon C. Butler, Arthur D. Odell, Benjamin Schachter, Marvin Darach, and myself.

In Dr. Marrian's obituary which Saul L. Cohen wrote for the Welcome Unit for the history of medicine, he included an anecdote which reflected Marrian's keen sense of humor. "After he (Marrian) had returned from a meeting of the American Society of Biological Scientists held in Detroit *circa* 1934, I (Cohen) asked him what was the most important thing he had learned at the meeting, and (Dr. Butenandt had described at these meetings the structure of the first androgen-androsterone) he replied, 'I learned that the only difference between Mae West and Clark Gable is 3 double bonds and 1 methyl group' (the difference in structure between estrone and androsterone!)."

Saul Cohen was Guy Marrian's first graduate student. His home was in Brandon, Manitoba. Together they developed the colorimetric Kober reaction for measuring the estrogen content of urine. They found that the estrogen excretion grew as a function of length of pregnancy and isolated estriol glucuronide in pure condition from late pregnancy urine. The process required the concentration of many gallons of pregnancy urine. Saul reported that he never had difficulty getting a seat on the street car no matter how crowded it was. The pungent odor of the urine concentrates clung to him tenaciously.

There was always a free exchange of ideas. For example, Gord Butler noted a Japanese paper describing an enzyme which hydrolyzed β-glucuronide linkages. Subsequently, Dr. Marrian asked me to prepare some of this enzyme to be tested for its ability to hydrolyze urinary estrogen glucuronides. I agreed and found myself wondering about the biochemical role of this enzyme in the body. This led to my doing my Ph.D. thesis on β-glucuronidase (4,5,6) and subsequently to publishing papers on this topic for thirty-six years in the interval from 1937-1973.

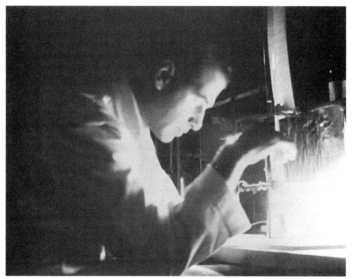

Titrating glucuronic acid released from substrate by β-glucuronidase - Bill Fishman

The camaraderie amongst Dr. Marrian's students was an important feature in providing a balance to the lives of the graduate students. Not only was there always light banter but, at night one could hear loud singing of bar-room ballads which entertained those who had time to listen. On payday, there was always a dinner at a local restaurant and an extensive pub crawl afterwards. This definitely reduced job stress.

Professor A.M. Wynne was a polished middle-aged gentleman who usually wore a blue serge suit and white shirt and tie. He was very interested in music. He saw his role as a teacher and did not have ambitions to become a leading researcher. However, all students who trained with him acquired a sound understanding of enzymology. I was one of them.

The arrival of Marvin Darrach from the University of British

Columbia as a graduate student contrasted markedly with the circumstances which greeted me in 1935. Every week for two months prior to his coming, Molly Delamere related favorable news, e.g., Darrach was one of the best qualified graduate students; he was accepted by Dr. Marrian who was very excited by the prospect of Darrach doing his Ph.D. thesis with him; he was a talented violinist; Dr. Wasteneys had succeeded in getting him into Toc H house, a residence of a fraternity character, etc., etc. Darrach was a handsome blue-eyed dark-haired man with charm, and for a while it seemed like he was the knight on the white horse. The reality though was that the White Horse (whiskey) was riding the knight. While under the influence, he "stood-up" Dr. Marrian who had scheduled an important experiment with Marvin. The "fire-works" which followed eventually led to Darrach taking a leave of absence. He finished his thesis some years later than he expected, after Dr. Marrian had moved to Edinburgh.

The graduate students treated alcohol with great respect and expertise. The laboratory grade of alcohol was 95% pure with 5% impurities and water. We took turns purifying the alcohol— first, it was exposed to pellets of pure sodium hydroxide—then it underwent fractional distillation with the ethanol containing fraction collected at the appropriate boiling point. At most, a liter of this absolute alcohol was recovered. When mixed with fruit juice it acquired the name "rain in the face". This potion was reserved for truly important celebrations

MY GRADUATE STUDIES AT TORONTO

Although the ability of β-glucuronidase to hydrolize urinary steroid glucuronides was prized by the steroid biochemists in the Marrian laboratory, my curiosity was directed to the possible role of the enzyme *in vivo*. It would be necessary to measure minute amounts of enzyme in tissues in animals whose biosynthesis of glucuronides had been enhanced.

It was possible to measure minute amounts of enzyme by lengthening the incubation period to seventy-two hours. The enzyme digests were saturated with the substrate of the enzyme leading to a linear release of glucuronic acid whose reducing power was measured by a modified Miller and Van Slyke ceric sulfate method. But how was the enzyme to be released from the tissue?

I designed tissue minihomogenizers (see figure below) powered by a pressured air stream. With a bank of six of these homogenizers the noise generated was excessive so they were

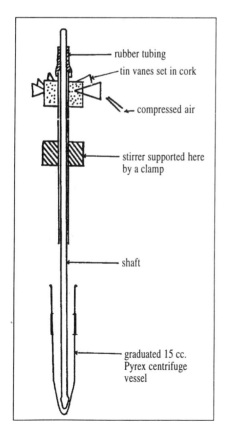

The Fishman Tissue
Minihomogenizer (ref. 7)

A solid glass rod is fitted with a short length of glass tubing inserted into the center of a cork into which tin vanes have been attached. This assembly when subjected to compressed air rotates freely on a glass tube supported by a rubber stopper clamped to a stand. The end of the solid glass rod is molded to fit the contours of a Pyrex graduated centrifuge tube. Fresh tissue (5-50 mg) is introduced into the bottom of the Pyrex centrifuge tube along with the required amount of buffer plus a small amount for rinsing. After a few minutes of homogenization the centrifuge tube is removed along with washings and centrifuged. The volume is recorded and aliquots of the supernatant removed for enzyme assay.

mounted in a chemical hood which could be closed off by a sliding door. This tissue homogenizer preceded the electrically-powered Potter-Elvehjem homogenizer which was widely used in biochemical tissue studies and cost approximately 1000% more.

The most interesting result was the reduction in the level of mouse uterine β-glucuronidase on castration and its restoration by the subsequent injection of estrogenic hormone. This triggered a decades-long exploration of hormonally-induced enzyme changes, the most significant of which has been the androgen-induction of mouse kidney β-glucuronidase activity.

It was forty-seven years later that I learned that my performance had generated praise from my mentor, Dr. Marrian. Thus, I was protected from acquiring a "swelled head." In January, 1937, in a letter to Saul Cohen, Dr. Marrian wrote the following:

> "Fishman is studying 'glucuronidase', at first simply as an enzyme and then will apply it to certain obvious oestrin problems. He is shaping up really well. He seems to have a remarkable flair for planning his experiments in a logical manner and he is a beautiful laboratory worker."

My work on β-glucuronidase was reported in three papers (4,5,6) in the *Journal of Biological Chemistry* under sole authorship. Dr. Marrian declined co-authorship because he felt that he had not contributed materially to the effort. So right from the beginning, I had achieved independence and graduated three years later with a Ph.D. in Biochemistry.

The "rite of passage" for a budding scientist is the presentation of one's research work to one's peers at a national meeting. In 1938, the American Society of Biological Chemistry was holding its annual meeting in Baltimore under the auspices of the Federation of American Societies for Experimental Biology with

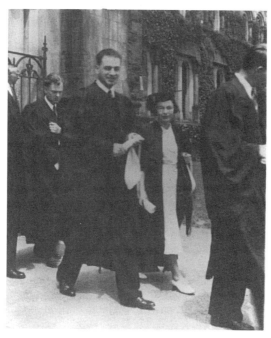

Bill with the Ph.D. diploma on graduation from the University of Toronto, 1939

an attendance of 2,000 scientists. Dr. Marrian had me submit an abstract of my work on ß-glucuronidase which was accepted for oral presentation. He and Mrs. Marrian motored to Baltimore with myself as the graduate student passenger. In Baltimore, my mind was most occupied with a rendezvous with Lillian Waterman, the future Lil Fishman, who had taken a train from New York to see me. Somehow I arrived at the lecture hall just as my paper was being announced. I strode to the podium, gave my lantern slides to the projectionist while at that very moment Dr. Marrian was rising to inform the chair of my absence. I am told that my presentation was excellent and that Dr. Marrian did recover rapidly from the anxiety he had experienced. Although Lil and I had corresponded over a year, the day in Baltimore was the third day we actually visited with each other. It confirmed our deep mutual interest and affection.

CHAPTER 5

MY WIFE

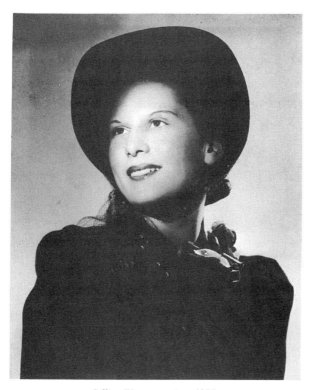

Lillian Waterman circa 1937

Lillian Waterman was born in Calgary, Alberta on April 28, 1915, the second daughter of Charles and Ethel Waterman of Trochu, Alberta. Charles was the third child of Sholom and Chaiah Waterman born in Suceava, Romania, where the family had operated an inn and distillery. In 1900, he immigrated first to New York and from there to Montreal ending up finally on a homestead land option near Trochu, Alberta. He and his brothers broke the land and planted wheat for their first crop. Charles became a successful farmer and married Ethel Guttman, the daughter of a neighboring farmer. Because Ethel was so industrious in the male Guttman household, Mr. Guttman made Charles wait five years before he would permit them to marry.

Charles and Ethel's family included in addition to Lillian, an older sister, Freda, a younger brother David and younger sister, Phyllis. As the children were reaching school age, the family moved to Calgary in order to join the Jewish community, and to provide the children an opportunity for a Hebrew education. While still operating the farm, Charles started a hardware import-export business out of his house. This grew into the now highly regarded and successful Western Canada Importers Company in Calgary currently managed by David Waterman.

Lillian was an excellent student and entered the Freshman class at the University of Alberta in Edmonton in 1931. She chose to follow the curriculum for a basic science-loaded bachelors degree in home economics. Her real interest, however, was in Biochemistry and to her surprise on graduation she was accepted as a graduate student at Columbia University's distinguished department of biochemistry. The reasons why Lillian turned down her great opportunity at Columbia do reflect the commonly-held attitudes of the times. Her family and others worried that a commitment to a higher science degree at a distant University would greatly reduce her chances of marriage. The academic climate promised no future for a woman in science although she was one of the leaders of her class. Everyone who graduated with her was successful in locating an accredited hospital for an internship in dietetics except Lil. Could it have been antisemitism? Finally, she volunteered to work in the dietary department of the Calgary General Hospital for one year, while continuing her search for an accredited internship. Later she was accepted without reservation by Montefiore Hospital, New York, in their dietitian training program.

When her Aunt Bessie Waterman saw Lil after she had finished her final examinations she was disturbed by her wan tired appearance. She invited Lil to have a vacation at her home in Saskatoon for a few weeks. About 60 miles from Saskatoon was Lake Manitou, a mineral water lake at Watrous. During the summer it was a meeting place of younger and older members of Western Canada Jewry. One day Lil was enjoying an afternoon with a girlfriend on the beach when I stopped to say hello. My appearance was not attractive at all. I had not shaved for three days and wore a black dusty sweater... but we found we had a lot to talk about. We agreed to meet at the dance hall that night.

Imagine my chagrin because she failed to recognize me when I appeared shaven and dressed in shirt and tie. As she was wearing rubber-soled shoes, our attempts to dance were futile and short-lived. However, we went for a walk and I found her to be very interested in my work and opinions of biochemistry. We agreed to write to each other.

We were actually in each others' company for five and a half days spread over two years of communication by letter before we became engaged. To some extent, my role models in this process were Gord and Jean Butler, who enthusiastically urged me to marry Lil. They were getting along on very little money but they were happy. The future of new scientists was very cloudy then for us all.

Our engagement was announced in Calgary on December 31, 1938 and this mutual commitment motivated Lil to come to Toronto and learn more about this guy who was planning to marry her. Without her parents' approval, she travelled to Toronto and became the roommate of the sister of a close friend of mine. However, she was bored and so I obtained permission for Lil to work with me in the laboratory. She attended departmental teas and entered into graduate student life. In the laboratory she prepared a biosynthetic substrate from the urine of rabbits previously fed menthol by stomach tube. This product was used for years afterwards. Finally, she typed my Ph.D. dissertation.

The affection with which Lil and I were held by the Staff was evidenced by their presentation to us of a wedding present: a silver plated casserole dish which had been designed and beautifully crafted by a silversmith.

In 1938, Professor Marrian accepted the Professorship of Medical Chemistry at the University of Edinburgh and invited me to apply for a Research Fellowship of the Royal Society of Canada. If I were successful in getting the award, I would do my post-doctoral study in Edinburgh. I was successful. This was an important milestone.

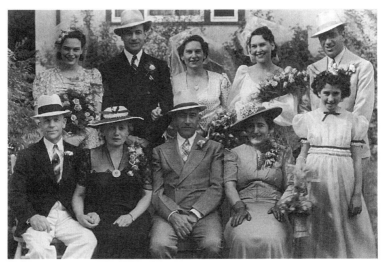

The Wedding Party, August 6, 1939. Back row (l. to r.) Phyllis Waterman, Bill Fishman, Lil Fishman, Freda Waterman, Saul Fishman; Front row - Charles Waterman, Ethel Waterman, Abraham Fishman, Goldie Fishman, Isobel Fishman

The future looked bright on graduation in June 1939. I was marrying Lil on August 6 and had saved enough money to buy us two return tickets on the Cunard Line from U.S. to U.K. To top all this, the stipend of the award was 1500 Canadian dollars and this would support us for one year. We would tour the continent also. There was little doubt in my mind that this was the first step of an academic career which ordinarily would be unfolding with predictable milestones ahead. Not so!

At this juncture, we will devote the rest of this chapter to the different roles Lil assumed in our life partnership even though reference to them is made in subsequent chapters.

In her training at the Montefiore, Sinai and New York hospitals, she was challenged by unexpected events. For example, she worked on the tuberculosis wards at Montefiore and was faced daily with seriously ill patients. At the New York Hospital which is affiliated with the Cornell University Medical School, she was a clinical dietician and was rotated from one floor to another. In addition she taught the nurses-in-training nutrition. In the course of this period in New York, she acquired managerial and administrative skills which equipped her to a large extent for the challenges which lay ahead.

Beginning with her initiation in Toronto of the stomach-tubing procedure for rabbits biosynthesizing menthol glucuronide, she showed an aptitude for learning new analytical techniques, organizing her experiments and developing original interpretations. So in Winston-Salem she prepared the synthetic diets deficient in choline which were fed to rats along with supplements of choline, ethanolamine and serine by stomach tube. Although she did no laboratory work from 1943 through 1949, in Boston, she set up the Pap stain technology for a collaborative study with a gynecologist, Dr. S. C. Kasdon. In addition, she was more than equal to the task of doing Microkjeldahl nitrogen analysis using the Parnas-Wagner apparatus. (Coincidentally, the co-inventor, Dr. Richard Wagner, a refugee from Nazi-Germany, joined the department of pediatrics at Tufts Medical School. He became our pediatrician. In Austria he was famous as the one who introduced insulin as the treatment for diabetes in the Kindersclinik in the late 1920's.)

With the arrival of our third offspring, Daniel Lewis in 1953, Lil devoted herself to the needs of the family until 1968. By then Joel and Nina were in college and Daniel was in High School. So at age 52, Lil enrolled at Boston University's department of education in the Master's degree program. Her goal was to earn the Master of Science Education degree and then to become a high school science teacher. It was a struggle. She had to acquire another general chemistry course as a prerequisite which she did by attending night classes at Harvard University extension. She studied embryology with pre-med students at Boston University. Finally, for her thesis requirement she polled students at the Driscoll elementary and junior high school on their TV viewing preferences and total hours in front of the TV. This original project was to be repeated over the years by many other analysts and commentators. Her practice training was performed at the Sharon high school some distance west of Boston. To add to her intellectual growth, she took Harvard courses in Italian. However, fate stepped in!

There was a health crisis in the family. It was me! I became a patient at the New England Medical Center hospital with a high fever and a perianal abscess. With the surgeon's assurance that I would be fine after the abscess was lanced, I consented to the surgery. The stay in the hospital was an ordeal with my large intestine and rectum being plugged by the huge amounts of Barium I swallowed and was given via rectum. The doctor's goal was to arrive at a diagnosis. Three additional operations failed to result in complete healing. It was not till 1985 that my problem was diagnosed as Crohn's disease.

Back in 1967, I urged Lil to return to the research lab as she was needed to meet the problems I was unable to deal with and to serve as the communication link to the staff. Besides she had real ability as a researcher, a career which would be more rewarding, in my opinion, than high school teaching. She agreed and the laboratory benefitted greatly.

With her strong determination and competence she mastered in a very short time a number of techniques which were indispensable for the research program. These included Sephadex gel column preparation and use for enzyme purification, tissue culture techniques and rabbit immunization and antibody production methodology and gel electrophoresis. In addition she became proficient in the enzyme histochemistry and immunochemistry of the alkaline phosphatase isozymes.

These were not simply technical exercises but were components to approach significant research problems, culminating in Lil's winning senior authorship on a paper (8) published in *Cancer Research*, 1976. It was a report on the developmental phase expression of placental alkaline phosphatase, this term heat-stable isozyme appears towards the end of the first trimester, increasing exponentially through the remainder of gestation. She solved the problem of polyacrylamide gel electrophoresis of high molecular weight aggregates of alkaline phosphatases by including the detergent, Triton x-100 both in the sample and in the gel. She was the sole author of this research report (9).

A contribution equally important to her efforts in the science arena was her extending warm hospitality to not only the laboratory staff but particularly the post-doctoral students from abroad. This would take the form of the annual picnic at Stage Fort park in Gloucester, the Thanksgiving dinner at the Fishmans, the Christmas party and New Year's day reception. The wives of the Japanese students would visit her on Friday afternoons not only to socialize but to improve their conversational English.

This warm personal interest in the Staff and visitors has continued without interruption to the present. Lil and I now host a quarterly reception for the new post-doctoral students and visiting scientists. This is the opportunity for Dr. Ruoslahti, the

President, to meet them as a group. In addition, Lil has organized an Alumni Association made up of former research staff members.

This chapter cannot end without an account of Lil's participation in communal life in Boston. She became Chairman of Education of Boston's Hadassah and organized a number of lectures by world-famous scholars such as Nahum Glatzer, and Rabbi Gold. In addition she was a member of Mr. Harris' select group of students studying the words of the prophet Jeremiah. She was an activist to get a permit from the Commonwealth of Massachusetts for a Public Education TV channel. The group was successful and Channel 2 was born in Boston.

In our last ten years in Boston, every week-end we would travel to Savory's Pond near Plymouth and enjoy our small cottage. I was able to clear enough land for us to put in a small garden, which produced prodigious amounts of cucumbers, tomatoes and onions. This was our best medicine for the stress in our lives.

OUR CHILDREN

Joel Shulem Fishman was born on May 4, 1943 in Winston-Salem North Carolina. Two years later the family moved to Chicago and in 1948, to Boston. His early education benefitted from the high scholastic standards of the Brookline schools, where he was attracted to the study of History. He also received a Hebrew education. Our six weeks in Japan opened the world beyond Boston to Joel and this partially motivated him to seek a career in history. His hobby in high school was photography which later became a life-long occupation. He received his B.A. from Tufts University in History and French and a Ph.D. from Columbia in Modern European History. His thesis, **Diplomacy and Revolution: The London Conference of 1830 and the Belgian Revolt**, was published in 1988 in Amsterdam.

During his doctoral studies, he won a Fulbright scholarship to study in Utrecht, Holland and after graduation, he spent three years in Amsterdam as a guest of the State Institute for War Documentation. There he carried out research and published on the history of Dutch Jewry in the Postwar era.

Returning to the USA, he found no employment opportunity in History. But there was something of the Fishman/Waterman pioneer spirit which motivated him to immigrate to Israel and to make his future there. He met his wife-to-be, Rivkah Duker, at a Columbia University reunion, and they were married on June 10, 1975.

Joel's career in Israel has been one of a photojournalist. Rivkah is a historian of the Roman and Byzantine periods and lectures both at Hebrew University and the Institute for Holy Land Studies. They have three children, Shammai Simcha, Rachel Malka, and Moshe Benjamin.

Nina Esther Fishman arrived in Winston-Salem two years after Joel on May 23, 1945 and enlivened our travel from Winston-Salem to Chicago. We were very pleased to have a daughter. She attended elementary and grade schools and Brookline High School, as well as Congregation Kehillath Israel's Hebrew education program. She was a top student who relished English literature. After two years at Boston University, she went to Reed College in Portland, Oregon to finish her B.A. in English literature. On her return to Boston, she completed her Master's degree in Education at Boston University.

She started in the Sommerville School System, Boston, as a specialist designing curricula for pre-school children. Her project was successful but with the loss of government grant support, she left the school education arena. Instead she took a position with a big insurance company to organize a training program for the insurance sales force.

This event set the course of her career from that time on. It led to the establishment of her own business as consultant on executive training and quality control. She lists NYNEX corporation and Bell Laboratories as her major clients. In 1992, she was married to Alan T. Attridge;, a business consultant and together they have created a start-up company, Natural Feast, Inc. which produces wheat-free food products for individuals with celiac disease.

Daniel Lewis Fishman was born in Boston on July 18, 1953 and also traveled the same educational route through the Brookline Schools and Kehillath Israel's program.

His higher education was interrupted by our move to California. At that time he had completed the first two undergraduate years at Tufts University.

Recognizing that his help was badly needed to get the Foundation started, he drove out to La Jolla in September 1976. The three of us were living, breathing and planning all day long into the night, the course of the La Jolla Cancer Research Foundation. Dan filled many roles until the Foundation could afford to hire full-time employees. For two years he was the director of Public Relations at LJCRF. However, he was most interested in journalism and photography and resumed his education at San Diego State University from which he graduated with a Bachelor's degree with distinction in Journalism and Advertising.

His great love as in the case of his older brother turned out to be photography. He specializes in event and fine portraiture photography and operates Flash Studios in Los Angeles.

CHAPTER 6

THE EDINBURGH EXPERIENCE

After a short honeymoon on Lake Wapta in the Canadian Rockies we travelled by train to New York. There we visited the World Fair and relatives and embarked on the Queen Mary where we found our cramped stateroom on D-deck. It was only then that we began to pay attention to the news of war clouds gathering over Europe. As we approached the continent of Europe, the ship was "blacked-out" and the ship's sailors were scrutinizing the waters for evidence of submarines.

We docked at Southampton and I thought I had ascertained how our new luggage packed with our wedding gifts was to be labeled for transfer to Edinburgh. A week after our luggage failed to arrive, we had the railroad officials track it down. It was still on the platform at Waterloo Station where we had failed to claim it and transfer it to the Edinburgh line. This is a testimonial to the honesty of the British and to the naiveté of the newlyweds.

In London we made our way to Gord and Jean Butler's apartment near Soho. We learned that Jean and their young son departed earlier to the country and that London was preparing for bombing and gas attacks by the German Luftwaffe. We spent that night with Gord and took the first train to Edinburgh.

In Edinburgh, we found Dr. and Mrs. Marrian preparing for the onset of war. The house was being "blacked-out"—we all were supplied with gas masks—the Marrian children had been evacuated to the countryside. The Marrians asked Lil and me to stay with them till we could find a place of our own. However, when Mrs. Marrian left for the country, Lil suddenly found herself in charge of the household, a role which was not expected nor welcomed.

One hour after Prime Minister Winston Churchill made Britain's declaration of war on Germany, the air raid alarm was sounded. Although no enemy planes were sighted then, this experience motivated us to start digging an air raid shelter immediately.

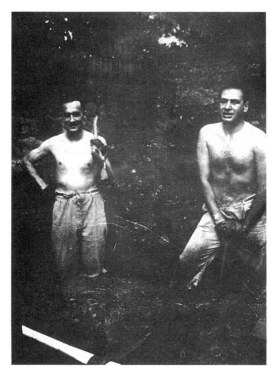

Bill Fishman and Guy Marrian digging an air raid shelter on
September 3, 1939 in Edinburgh, Scotland

We had an important decision to make—do we stay or do we go back? Another post-doctoral student of Marrian's from Toronto had arrived the previous week and as the war clouds gathered, departed quickly to Sweden, a neutral country. It seemed to us that if we lacked the will to proceed along the path we had committed ourselves to, this would not augur well for meeting the many challenges which lay ahead. We decided to stay the year—another milestone!

SCIENCE DURING WAR TIME

The "new buildings" of the Edinburgh University's medical school were built at the turn of the century to duplicate the architecture of an Italian monastery. The stone walls were five feet thick and the windows were recessed two feet to reduce the glare of the sun (in Edinburgh, the sun never glares, especially in winter). The rooms for the laboratories were of a reasonable size except for the ceilings which were 18 feet high. The walls were greyish black from the soot accumulation over many years. My first task was to wash down the walls and paint them. I could not reach the ceiling by standing on the lab benches. The animal rooms were in the basement of another building across the quadrangle.

The department was staffed by the Professor and Head, Dr. G. F. Marrian and Dr. and Mrs. Steadman. Younger staff included Dr. Miekeljohn, G. Levvy and Borthwick supported by the laboratory manager, Mr. Rankeilor.

The ambiance in the Edinburgh laboratory was quite a bit different than in Toronto. The Professor occupied and enjoyed a position much more exalted and powerful than the head of a department in Canada. The "Chief" exercised full control and held everyone's attention. Dr. Marrian really enjoyed his privileged position.

As Lil volunteered to work with me in the laboratory, it was possible to rapidly undertake experiments, the results of which were published (10) under our two names in the *Journal of Biological Chemistry* in 1944. We reported on the first induction of enzyme activity by estrogenic hormones. The mice needed attention seven days a week and a full schedule of experiments was initiated.

It was not all work and no play, however. We were able to attend several good theatrical productions such as Eugene

O'Neill's "Desire under the elms" with John Gielgud. We became good friends of Doctors Pepi and Joe Adler, refugees from Hitler's Vienna, Sara and J. M. Robson and Dr. Michaelis. Joe Adler and J. M. Robson were on the staff of the Pharmacology department. A visiting scientist at that time was the Nobel prize winner-to-be Dr. H. J. Mueller who later pursued his genetic research at the University of Indiana. He had the foresight to suggest that it was most important to establish the chemical structure of the gene.

We found that class distinctions were exercised by the senior faculty at the University. When the Chief of Pharmacology was leaving to join the Armed Services, all the Jewish members of the Faculty were excluded from his farewell party.

The following recollections describe snapshots of our lives in Edinburgh.

I had to leave Edinburgh to present a paper at Oxford University just when we were moving to our apartment at 46 Marchmont Circle. Lil boarded a streetcar at night with our last few possessions in her hands. Although the fare was twopence, she was able to come up with a penny, a hapenny and two farthings. The conductor took the money, opened Lil's hand and returned the fare. When she left the trolley, she noticed that a policeman was following her some 100 feet behind her. He left once she had entered the apartment house. Silently, he was providing a protective escort during the blackout. The wonderful Scots!

The days were very short and very cold in the winter because Edinburgh is on the same latitude as Peace River in northern Alberta. I wore longjohns, wool socks, sweater, a thick Harris Tweed 3-piece suit, wool scarf and a wool coat, all of which prevented me from freezing. There was very little difference between the temperatures indoors and outdoors as there was no central heating. Before ones' hands could be thawed out to do the pipeting, we turned on all the Bunsen gas burners and electric hot plates. One morning I smelled the smoke of burning wool. It was due to my back being warmed too much by the gas burner flame.

The apartment we lived in had a fireplace in each room. The one in the kitchen heated water which found its way to the cold metal zinc bathtub when the bathtub tap was turned. The fact is that the ice cold zinc bathtub absorbed all the heat from the water and one spent a very short time in the tub in order not to be chilled.

Before going to sleep, we took turns placing a hot water bottle under the bed sheets at the foot of the bed. Next, one of us would leap into bed and assume an immobile position with our feet on the hot water bottle; the other areas of the bed were very cold. Once the combination of hot water bottle heat and one's body heat had reduced the shivering, the other spouse would quickly make a rapid entry and assumed a position as close as possible to the original occupant. Eventually, after the shivering stopped we fell asleep.

Lil's first experience lighting a fire in the kitchen fireplace was an ordeal. There was not enough kindling, she did not know how the drafts worked, the coal was wet. After using up a box of matches and after expending a great deal of persistence, and after many trials and errors, success finally came.

The Scottish butcher shop was interesting. On display were carcasses of animals unfamiliar to us, skinned rabbit we learned later, as well as pheasants. At one dinner we were asked if we liked hare, the main dish... it was a bit of a shock... after having seen them at the butcher's, but ate it anyway, disguising our true feelings.

In the lab at lunch time Mr. Borthwick was munching on his shepherd's pie while he read the local newspaper, *The Scotsman*. Aloud he commented quietly - hmm! the Jerrys have sunk several ships in the Atlantic - Well, the U.S. doesn't seem to be concerned! - then he jumped up and ran up to each of us and exclaimed loudly

- "They have found Wallace's sword!" To a Scotsman this was the news item of the year.

We started a Victory garden which our neighbors later inherited.

Several reasons combined to decide us to return to Canada in May of 1940. There was no opportunity for me to do war research in U.K.; the prospects of my pursuing a scientific career in Britain were non-existent and our parents were very anxious for us to return to Canada in view of the danger to Jews if Hitler's forces ever were to invade Britain.

This decision was reinforced when we listened in astonishment and disbelief to the news of German paratroopers landing in Holland and the progress of panzer divisions into that country. Luckily we still had the return portion of our Cunard Line tickets. The process of booking the journey, closing up the apartment, settling our accounts, saying farewell and taking an overnight train to Liverpool took 48 hours.

We found ourselves passengers on a small Cunard ship with people who had experienced the defeat at Dunkirk and others who were refugees from Hitler's regime. Accompanying us on the two week zig-zag journey was a British battle ship which was carrying Queen Wilhelmina and her family from Holland and all the gold of the Bank of France. With this protection the danger of submarine attacks was greatly reduced.

Landing in Montreal, I sought out Professor J. B. Collip at McGill University and declared my immediate availability for war research. His reply was that the Canadian government was waiting for the British to define their needs and he could not predict when this would happen.

Returning to Toronto, Dr. Wasteneys proposed that I spend the second year of my fellowship at any good biochemistry department outside Canada that would accept me. Purely from my understanding of the biochemical literature, the two premier laboratories in the United States at that time were Dr. V. du Vigneaud's at Cornell University Medical College in New York and Dr. C. A. Elvehjem's at the University of Wisconsin. I chose du Vigneaud and he accepted me sight unseen. This was another important milestone.

CHAPTER 7

NEW YORK, NEW YORK

Dr. du Vigneaud was a tall strong man with tremendous drive, great organizing ability and ambition to excel. He had just been appointed to Cornell from Georgetown University in Washington, D.C. His laboratory was credited with discovering - methyl group transfer from choline to methionine. With him came his graduate students, new staff and foreign post-doctoral students.

How did he keep track of all the research he directed? There were projects on the isolation and characterization of pituitary pitocin and oxytocin, on the use of the deuterium isotope as a molecular marker of methyl group transfer, on the isolation and characterization of biotin, et cetera et cetera. The pioneer studies on the pituitary hormones earned him a Nobel Prize, later.

His co-workers would communicate their findings and questions on green slips to his secretary and when du Vigneaud thought there was a need for discussion, you would be summoned. You would find him stretched out on a black leather sofa and the question on his lips was always the same, "Where were we in our thinking on your project?" After you presented its history, a discussion would result and new objectives were defined. There was an economy of conversation.

Scientists in the laboratory at that time later became well-known figures in biochemistry.

First there was Fritz Lipmann, a German refugee, who would shuffle absentmindedly into his lab in mid-morning and sit on a high stool for at least an hour deep in thought. He then leapt into a frenzy of activity, sacrificing a pigeon, dissecting out the breast muscles, mincing them and introducing measured amounts into Warburg vessels which were then fitted with manometers mounted in sets of six onto a Warburg bath. These were the experiments which supported his concept of high energy phosphate which eventually led to the award to him of the Nobel Prize.

Next there was Klaus .Hofmann, a master at organic chemistry who trained with the world-famous Swiss scientists Professors Reichstein and Ruzicka. He cracked the biotin problem and went on to chair and direct the University of Pittsburgh protein chemistry lab.

Also, Dean Burk and Richard Winzler shared a laboratory with Dr. Lippman. Dean Burk was responsible with Lineweaver in formulating the Lineweaver-Burk equations which are the basis of classical enzymologic kinetics. Later, Burk engaged in a bitter defense of Otto Warburg's view of the etiology of cancer. Dick Winzler discovered sialic acid in the circulation and became well-known in the carbohydrate field.

Finally, Mildred Cohn was assembling one of the first mass spectrometers with which to measure deuterium isotope recovered from pure metabolites. However, until this instrument was completed we used the cumbersome, demanding "falling drop" densitometric method which was less sensitive. She was my coworker on a paper (11) we published on acetate for conjugation reactions coming from one metabolic pool. Mildred Cohn was a pioneer in isotope studies such as this one, became a famous scientist and is now an emeritus member of the Fox Chase Cancer Center.

Imagine my feelings of inadequacy to be in the company of scientists in my age group who were so much more experienced and talented than I was. It was a great learning experience, made even more valuable by contacts with faculty in other departments. These included Dr. Papanicalaou who devised the "Pap" test for cervical cancer, Dr. Ephraim Shorr, a clinical endocrinologist and Dr. E. A. Kabat who became a famous immunologist. The seminars at Cornell featured some of the leaders in biochemical research who escaped Hitler's Germany. These included Otto Meyerhoff, Rudolph Schoenheimer, Heinrich Waelsch, Zacharias Dische and others. Schoenheimer was a handsome intense scientist who introduced the use of radioactive isotopes of carbon and hydrogen into the study of intermediary metabolism.

LIFE IN THE BIG APPLE

In 1940, New York still had many of its early life style and experiences intact - such as the pushcart vendors on Second Avenue - 5¢ subway fares - and a high cost of living.

The stipend of the second year award of my fellowship was reduced to $1200 due to the relative weakness of the Canadian dollar. How were we to live in New York on $100 a month? With difficulty! First we located a one-room studio several blocks from Cornell for $35 a month. Then we got a bed, a second-hand carpet and a minimum of furniture. Our steamer trunk served as a dresser. We never bought a newspaper or an ice cream cone.

However, Lil found employment as a dietitian at Mount Sinai Hospital first and then later at New York Hospital which is the teaching hospital of Cornell University School of Medicine. On her return home from her first day at work, she found that I had bought a case of Bock beer and a newspaper. This was a happy day!

Jones Beach beckoned to these two land-locked souls in the big city. One summer day, we arrived by subway at the beach, bringing a picnic lunch and joining a crowd stretched out on the sand and swimming in the surf. The sky was overcast but the sun was warm. Lil, who is fair-skinned, was severely sun-burned, while I am darker-skinned, and was only mildly affected. The next morning found me putting ointment and bandages on the burned areas and helping Lil into her uniform. She was insistent on reporting for duty. I now had a wife with freckles.

A U.S. presidential election occurred in 1940 - Franklin Roosevelt versus Wendell Wilkie. We attended an election eve party at the Winzler apartment as observers. The arguments between supporters of each of the two candidates were spirited and confrontational. Roosevelt won.

The Borek's extended their hospitality to us. Ernest Borek was on the faculty at Columbia and at City College. His wife, née Minuetta Shumiatcher originally a Calgary friend of Lil's, was an accomplished pianist and composer. At their home we met other scientists which included David Rittenberg and Sune Bergstrom of Sweden. Our paths were to cross frequently.

WHERE NEXT?

As the spring of 1941 arrived, it became important that I find my next position as the Royal Society of Canada Fellowship would expire by September 1. I shared my concern with Dr. du Vigneaud. At the spring meeting of the Federation of American Societies for Experimental Biology, he was approached by Dr. Camillo Artom who was looking for an instructor in biochemistry. Dr. du Vigneaud gave me a good recommendation and I was hired. I was now on the first step of the academic ladder in a brand new Medical School in the middle of North Carolina. An important milestone!

CHAPTER 8

WINSTON-SALEM AND THE BOWMAN-GRAY SCHOOL OF MEDICINE

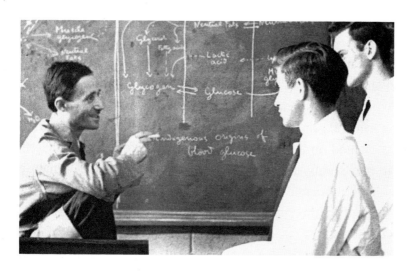

Professor Camillo Artom in discussion with medical students of the
Bowman-Gray School of Medicine, Winston-Salem, NC

Cami Artom was all of five feet in height, weighed less than 100 lbs., with eyes which though bright and gentle were profoundly astigmatic, and with his head cocked at an odd angle but with a warm heart and a fine intelligence. He had been a professor of biochemistry at the University of Palermo, Italy, where he had collaborated with Enrico Fermi in employing fats labeled with radioisotopic iodine to track their intermediary metabolism. This was another pioneering independent use of isotopes in biochemistry.

With the adoption by Mussolini of the restrictive, Jewish-persecution Nazi edicts, Dr. Artom could no longer hold his appointment at the University. He was recruited in 1939 to head the biochemistry department of Wake Forest College which was

located in eastern North Carolina. In 1941 Wake Forest College
Medical School became the Bowman-Gray School of Medicine
and it was established in Winston-Salem in the heart of the
Piedmont region. I joined the Faculty about one month before
the School opened and we were completely broke. Fortunately,
Dr. Artom advanced me $50 from my first paycheck.

The embryonic Bowman-Gray School of Medicine was
struggling fiscally and it was with great difficulty that it committed
an annual salary of $1800 to me. We did find a nice apartment at
Twin Castles Apartments, which were only a short distance from
the medical school. What saved our budget was a Victory Garden
we planted on the banks of a creek at the foot of Twin Castles.
We had plenty of water and used an opened large tomato can
with holes punched in the bottom for transferring the water from
a bucket to the plants. We were thrilled with the harvest of
cucumbers, onions, corn, radishes with which we were familiar
but especially with the okra, canteloupe and watermelon which
do not grow in Western Canada.

Dr. Artom was completely devoted to his research and the
medical students. In but a few months, the biochemistry lectures

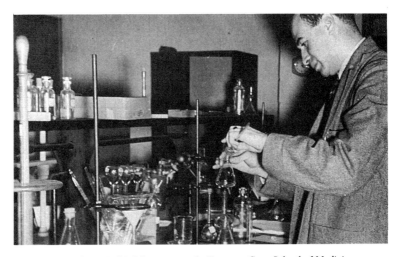

Bill Fishman in his laboratory at the Bowman-Gray School of Medicine

and laboratory exercises had to be organized and made ready for the first class of future doctors. My teaching experiences in Toronto stood me in good stead.

I was given full responsibility for the laboratory exercises and designed them so that the students could learn first-hand the principles which were clearly relevant to the practice of medicine. For example, the students performed glucose tolerance tests on each other. This involved drawing six samples of blood from each other at intervals after ingesting a concentrated glucose solution - measuring the blood glucose - plotting the results on paper - and discussing them in relation to diabetes. We had a limited supply of syringes and needles and this required a continuous cycling of the syringes and needles through manual washing and sterilization. On another occasion, the fasting subjects swallowed stomach tubes and after the residual gastric juice was removed, they were exposed in another room to the sight and smell of hamburgers being fried. This elicited a large amount of gastric juice. All specimens were analyzed for hydrogen ion concentration, and for various digestive enzymes—discussion related to gastric and duodenal ulcers.

The lectures were delivered for the most part by Dr. Artom. There was sometimes a problem in communication - Dr. Artom's English was his second language and he was surrounded by English spoken with a Southern accent. For example, when he was discussing conjugation mechanisms, he used the construction, "When molecule A is copulated with molecule B". He meant "coupled". This problem was solved when rather full texts of the lectures were made available to the students.

Opening day of the Bowman-Gray School of Medicine was witnessed by a unique faculty. Its most prominent member was the Professor of Medicine - Tinsley Harrison who brought with him, a distinguished Johns Hopkins researcher, Dr. Arthur Grollman. He had perfected the rat experimental model for inducing hypertension and the Dean believed that a cure was just about to be found in Grollman's laboratory. Other younger faculty were George Harrell, Frank Locke, Nash Herndon, and John R. Williams. In Physiology, Dr. Herbert Wells from Vanderbilt, Dr. William Govier and Dr. Max Little were the staff. Many of the clinical staff were prominent physicians in Winston-Salem such as Dr. Wingate Johnson and William H. Sprunt Jr. The Pathology Lab was headed by Dr. Robert P. Morehead and was a resource to the entire Piedmont region. Altogether about eighteen individuals formed the active faculty and perhaps eight of them were devoted to research.

The medical school had a very meager research budget and Dr. Artom personally approached the Dazian Foundation in New York for $1200 and received an award. It had not occurred to me to ask how much research money would be available when I was being interviewed for the position.

What would I be researching? I had considered extending the deuterium isotope acetylation studies to new areas and brought this to Dr. du Vigneaud's attention while at Cornell. He stated "Fishman, we gave you the ball to play with while you were here. When you leave, the ball stays here for your successor." (Interestingly, that ball did not receive a player ever after). My decision then was to work with Dr. Artom on his project on the biochemistry of liver phospholipids.

I learned a great deal from my association with Dr. Artom. Aside from the technical expertise which I acquired in preparing, fractionating and measuring liver lipids from rats maintained on synthetic diets rich in either choline, serine or ethanolamine, I was impressed with Artom's ability to harvest every piece of significant information from columns of data. This harvest was a consequence of intensive analysis, critical review of the limits of error in the analysis and the practicality of statistics and their limitations (12).

Lil became the unpaid volunteer dietitian to the rat colony. Groups of these animals were on the same choline-deficient diet but received equivalent amounts by stomach tube of saline solutions of either choline, ethanolamine or serine. After a few days we were surprised to find that only the serine cage now contained several dead rats. In showing these animals to the pathologist, Cami Artom asserted "These animals did not die because they were tired of living." Dr. Morehead reported necrosis of the proximal kidney tubules. This "serine injury" (13) has been referred to ever since in studies of nephrotoxic agents.

DECEMBER 7, 1941

We were listening to our transplanted Scottish Ferguson radio that Sunday afternoon and heard President Roosevelt's report of "the day that will live in infamy"—Pearl Harbor. The declaration of war against Japan and Germany followed soon afterwards.

The immediate consequence to the faculty was that a new freshman class was on board every nine months instead of at twelve month intervals and most of them were in uniform. They were all committed by the Navy and Army medical training programs to enter the armed services. We were teaching literally "around the clock." Rationing was instituted and we were now gardening more grimly than happily.

As a faculty member, I was presented with a career choice. I could enlist in the Medical Officers training corps, wear a military uniform, receive a salary greater than my current stipend, and graduate with an M.D. degree in three years. Several faculty made this choice. I decided to continue as an instructor in biochemistry and to focus on my research. I reasoned, perhaps that in the end the benefits of basic research would reach many more patients than an individual doctor could treat. It also seemed to me that after the M.D. training I would no longer be the same scientist after leaving the laboratory for three years and having to practice the art of medicine.

A DIAGNOSTIC PROBLEM! A BABY!

Lil was not feeling well in October of 1942 and went to see Dr. Grollman. He examined her and opined that she had a big growth in her pelvis. It was big indeed and grew eventually to a seven pound 11 ounce baby boy born on May 3, 1943. His name is Joel Shulem (the two names are those of our paternal grandparents). Life was never to be the same!

We were living in a small cottage on the outskirts of Winston-Salem at that time. Our neighbor operated a farm and was kind enough to permit us to put in a victory garden on an adjacent lot. Again, I was digging and together we succeeded in planting a garden some 50 feet by 150 feet in dimensions. The "manure" in this area was tobacco dust from the R.J. Reynolds Company and it helped make the red clay more porous. We harvested tremendous amounts of tomatoes, cucumbers, onions, okra, etc. and were especially excited about the yellow variety of tomatoes. Lil canned about 50 quarts of tomatoes for the winter months which were our source of vitamin C in the fall and winter.

The war in Europe affected us directly in several ways. Lil's brother had joined the Royal Canadian Air Force early in the war, my brother enlisted in the Canadian armed services, and many of our relatives and friends were already overseas in Britain preparing for D-day. In Austria, Lil's father's cousin, Irving Hopmeier and his family were refugees staying just a step ahead of the Gestapo secret Nazi police. Every effort was being made on this side of the Atlantic to obtain permission for them to immigrate to the U.S. or Canada. Just a few days after Lil and Joel returned from the hospital, I received a notice to appear before a committee of the State Department to testify in favor of a visa for the Hopmeiers. I went but encountered a cold negative decision. All through the war we sent medicines and food to the Hopmeiers. They made it to Spain, fought in the French underground, and survived the war. The war years were ones of anxiety, struggle and sacrifice for us all.

Several highlights of our lives in Winston-Salem from 1941-1945 follow.

-One of the medical students brought me a huge country ham as a present. I politely did not accept it as Lil and I don't eat ham in accordance with our tradition. Imagine our surprise when we were invited to the Artom's who served a country ham which they stated was a present from the same grateful student. We gorged on the yams, salad and bread but not the ham.

-A student happened to meet us at our primitive garden at the foot of Twin Castles. We offered him a bunch of vegetables which he gratefully accepted. He told us later that this was the only food in the house for himself and his sister's family that whole week. We were the recipients subsequently of a bench and stool which he had built himself.

-Lil became the President of the Irma Lindheim chapter of Hadassah whose main concerns were saving European Jewish children for Aliyah to what was then Palestine. She published a Newsletter, an activity which was to recur throughout her career. The Chapter organized their first Fundraiser Donor Banquet, the proceeds of which supported a room in the Mt. Scopus Hadassah Hospital. Her fundraising talents were also to emerge successfully at intervals for years ahead.

-One of our best medical students ended up in the hospital with a bad case of poison ivy poisoning. He was later to head the Duke Comprehensive Cancer Center as an outstanding surgeon, Dr. William Shingleton.

-Dr. Artom showed me a letter from Dr. Lewis at the University of Michigan's biochemistry department in which he listed Ph.D.

graduates who were looking for an academic position. One name only was identified as Jewish, presumably so that the prospective employer could be forewarned. "Equal Opportunity" was not a principle widely accepted at that time! The name was Dr. Eugene Roberts who was to become significant decades later in the life of the La Jolla Cancer Research Foundation.

After four years at Bowman-Gray, it was time to move on. Dr. Artom and I were managing very well to handle the teaching load and to produce a good number of significant publications. However, I felt that a limit had been reached in what I could achieve as the junior staff member. I hungered for a position where there was a community of active biochemists. There was also the financial needs of a growing family - Nina having arrived on May 23, 1945. My salary was now $3600 per annum while Dr. Artom's was $3900. Upward mobility in terms of compensation was at an end.

I explained to Dr. Artom my intention to explore opportunities elsewhere and if none materialized I would stay at Bowman Gray with him without limitation of time. He accepted gracefully but sadly saying "sometimes people get a divorce."

How was I to find another job? I wrote to all the chairmen of the biochemistry departments at universities, answered all the relevant advertisements in *Chemical and Engineering News* and waited and waited. Finally, the few replies that arrived included one from the Department of Surgery at the University of Chicago. This intrigued me as it would offer opportunities to do research on patients in a biochemical environment which included scientists such as Tom Gallagher, E. Guzman-Baron, Earl Evans, Konrad Bloch and others. The Chicago milestone was now at hand.

CHAPTER 9

CHICAGO AND THE UNIVERSITY OF CHICAGO, MY ENTRY INTO CANCER RESEARCH

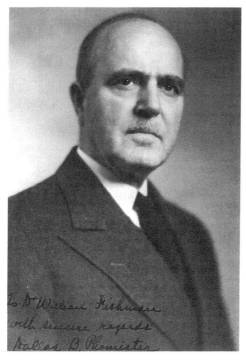

Professor Dallas B. Phemister, Chairman, Department of Surgery, University of Chicago - 1947

Dr. Dallas B. Phemister was the Chairman of the department of Surgery at the University of Chicago in 1945. With the introduction of the effective antibiotics, sulfanilamide and penicillin, during the war years, he saw that the Surgical Bacteriology Lab. of his department was becoming obsolete. Moreover, he was convinced that the problems which surgeons had to wrestle with could best be solved through biochemistry.

Accordingly he secured a grant from the O. S. Sprague Foundation out of which a salary of $5000 was available for a biochemist. The candidate also needed to be approved by Dr. Earl Evans of the Biochemistry department.

Dr. Phemister was a gracious gentleman. He had me stay at his home during the two days of interviews and treated me with every consideration.

He believed that a biochemist could solve all the research problems of the senior surgical staff and so I was interviewed by Dr. Charles B. Huggins (later a Nobel Laureate), Dr. Lester Dragstedt (vagotomy for gastric ulcer), Dr. Alex Brunschwig (exenterotomy in oncologic surgery), Dr. Adams (thoracic surgery) and Dr. Livingston (anesthesiology). Dr. Phemister himself was anxious to research post-operative anemia, a mysterious condition which afflicted patients even though their blood loss had been corrected by an adequate number of blood transfusions. My job was to assist all these surgeons in their research and, by the way, I was expected to do my own research as well. Then, almost as an afterthought, I was asked to manage the Surgical Chemistry lab. It was soon apparent that this facility which was indispensable for the surgeons to deal with pre- and post-operative situations was in a serious decline. I sensed that to turn the clinical laboratory around should be the first priority of my time and energy. I took the job and its many challenges. Before I left Chicago, there were close to a dozen technicians under my supervision.

I rolled up my sleeves and worked through every technique and established quality control procedures; became an expert with the use of the Van Slyke CO_2 manometric apparatus and recruited a staff of five. The surgeons were happy with the lab's performance.

However, the management of a clinical lab can have its emergency moments. As for example, on my return from a

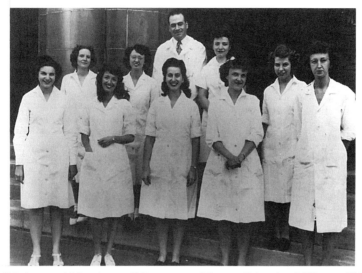

Bill Fishman and laboratory staff, Department of Surgery, University of Chicago - 1948

vacation in Canada, I was surprised to find that four of the five lab staff had left for one reason or another. Again, I rolled up my sleeves and the 18 hour days became the norm. The staff vacancies were filled and the analyses were completed on time.

The surgical residents interfaced with me on the research projects of their professors. Two quite different experiences illustrate the interaction.

Dr. J. Garrott Allen, Dr. Phemister's resident had very definite ideas of how to approach the problem of post-operative anemia. One day he presented me with three type-written, single spaced pages of analyses that I was to perform on blood, urine and feces of surgical patients. Items included the various porphyrins, iron balance, etc. How to deal with this?

My position was that this proposal was premature. One had to know which types of patients undergoing which surgical procedure entailing the loss of how many pints of blood would be the best candidates for the highly sophisticated protocol of analyses. I suggested that the next one hundred surgical patients be evaluated for this key information. It turned out that he was the one who had to collect the surgical dressings, wash them in a washing machine and measure the hemoglobin content in addition to keeping the detailed records. The project as Allan proposed never got off the ground much to my relief.

MY ENTRY INTO CANCER RESEARCH

Dr. A. John Anlyan was the resident on surgical pathology in 1946. Every day surgical specimens were carried past my laboratory to the surgical pathology lab. I had in the meanwhile returned to my research interest in β-glucuronidase, on which my last studies had been done in Edinburgh. However, in my first year in Chicago, I collaborated with Paul Talalay (then a second-year medical student) in generating a new rapid assay technique for β-glucuronidase (14). Paul was working in the laboratory of Dr. Charles Huggins who later received the Nobel Prize for his work on prostatic cancer. I was curious to find out what levels of β-glucuronidase activity were present in human cancer tissue. John Anlyan entered enthusiastically into this inquiry and provided the individual specimens and the histologic diagnoses. We found that the majority of tumor tissues expressed high levels of the enzyme as compared to adjacent non-cancerous tissue, an unexpected result as the accepted viewpoint was that cancer tissues showed diminished enzyme activity.

We had serious competition—to our concern—not from scientists in other institutions but from Charles Huggins in our own department. He was employing the rapid enzyme assay on the same surgical specimens that we were assaying. John became aware of this. We immediately sent a "Letter to the Editor" to the *Journal of Biological Chemistry* entitled "The presence of high β-glucuronidase activity in cancer tissue (15)." Before it was published I presented our results to the surgical group. Dr. Huggins stated then that they had given up their study of cancer tissues too soon because they had not been as "pertinaceous" as Dr. Fishman. Our discovery of the β-glucuronidase enrichment of human tumor tissue marked the origin of my interest in the cancer problem and its relevance to humans. This was to persist and grow for the rest of my life.

One day Dr. Huggins was next to me in the cafeteria line. He said to me, "Bill, you know you are a rival of mine." I was astounded as I never did picture myself at his level of achievement.

As for John Anlyan, he went on to academic appointments at Ohio State, Sloan-Kettering Institute and Yale University before initiating a successful practice in San Francisco as a cancer surgeon. His two brothers were outstanding physicians and Yale graduates. William Anlyan, a surgeon, became Dean of the medical school at Duke University. John expressed his appreciation to Yale with a bequest of $25,000,000, the largest single gift the institution had received. He was and is a remarkable human being.

My first experiences were with human cancer in contrast to the majority of biochemists in the cancer field. They were studying transplantable hepatomas in mice and rats primarily because these animals produced a large tumor mass in a short time. The excised tumor tissue was minced or homogenized and its respiration evaluated by the Warburg manometric procedure. The conceptual dogma (16) elaborated by Nobelist Otto Warburg was that tumors adopted a fermentation rather than an oxidation mechanism to produce chemical energy from carbohydrates and this was the cause of cancer. This view was to dominate cancer research from 1933 through to 1960 when elucidation of actual metabolic pathways with the use of isotopic markers failed to demonstrate Warburg's so-called defect in respiration.

Another experience was important in focusing my interest on the potential of enzyme histochemistry in my further studies. This was my collaboration with Dr. George Gomori who was a

Hungarian refugee working in thoracic medicine. He has been recognized as the major pioneer in the fashioning of histochemical techniques for the phosphatases. Such techniques make visible the sites in thin tissue sections which harbor the enzyme under investigation.

He suggested that I prepare by biosynthesis, the glucuronide of 2,4-dichloronaphthol which when hydrolyzed by the cancer cell β-glucuronidase would release the poorly soluble 2,4-dichloronaphthol. In the presence of an appropriate diazonium salt, a black dye would be deposited at the enzyme site. The glucuronide was isolated from the urine of rabbits after they were dosed with an emulsion of the naphthol. Shortly afterwards we applied this histochemical test to a suspension of cancer cells in an ascitic fluid of a cancer patient. We were excited to see a number of cells stained black but disappointed that other cancer cells were unstained. We did not continue the study. In retrospect, the failure was not in the technique but in our limited understanding of the variable enzyme expression of cancer cells. Dr. Gomori went on to make major contributions to histochemistry and is regarded as the founder of histochemistry in the West.

Living in Chicago in 1945-1948 presented many more challenges than the ones we encountered in the semi-rural city of Winston-Salem. We had arrived in Chicago after a harrowing journey by train as a consequence of torrential downpours of rain which caused long delays. We checked the children's cribs and baby carriage as baggage and so we were able to settle them down comfortably in the apartment we had rented. Our bed and furniture, however, did not arrive for two months because of war-time delays. We managed to sleep fitfully on cardboard placed on top of the springs of the Murphy bed (which folds into the wall when not in use).

Although Chicago was dubbed the windy city, it also could in the summertime be named the oppressive heat city and in the winter, as the cold windy city. One month of August we experienced twenty-one days of over 90°F weather. Our only relief was to walk to Lake Michigan close by and immerse ourselves in the water. In the long winter, Lil would be pushing the baby carriage with Nina in it and Joel struggling to climb aboard. Nina refused to wear mittens and cried because she was cold. To make ends meet, Lil, with the two kids in tow, made the rounds of the grocery stores to save pennies on food items.

Just after eighteen months when I felt I was managing all my responsibilities successfully and was looking forward to climbing the academic ladder at the University of Chicago, there was distressing news. Dr. Phemister was to retire in six months and he was to be succeeded by Dr. Lester Dragstedt. The climate turned from warm to cold and it was clear that there was no future for me at Chicago. This was yet another experience in my career where performance was not rewarded.

Dr. Earl Evans, the Chairman of the Biochemistry Department, helped me to see that the big picture held much hope for me. He explained that scientists belong to a world community, that I should find opportunity elsewhere and that I should not embitter myself at Chicago. In his department at the time was an able steroid biochemist, Dr. Tom Gallagher, who had taken a friendly interest in me. He appeared to enjoy my reports of incidents in which the aggressive surgical residents came out second best. He became my mentor in the ways to survive in the academic jungle and still retain one's integrity.

Opportunity did knock on my door! In 1948, the National Cancer Institute granted each medical school $25,000 per annum to develop and implement a program for the teaching of cancer to medical students. Up to that time, the students received in their senior year, fragmented cancer information usually in relation to diseases of different organs. There was no presentation of concepts of cancer biology and etiology. Tufts Medical School in Boston saw this grant as a way to attract research oncologists to their faculty without increasing the budget very much. Sloan-Kettering Memorial Institute in New York at that time was a leading cancer research center pioneering in steroid metabolism, chemotherapy, radiation therapy and surgery. Accordingly, Dr. Stuart Welch, the chief surgeon at Tufts approached Sloan-Kettering for an oncologist to head the cancer teaching program at Tufts.

Dr. Freddy Homburger was the choice. He was a graduate of the University of Geneva Medical School, had trained at Yale and at Harvard and was the Director of Clinical Investigation at Sloan-Kettering. He needed a basic scientist working in oncology to build the scientific base of the Cancer Research and Cancer Control Unit at Tufts. Dr. Gallagher recommended me to Dr. Konrad Dobriner who in turn brought my name to Dr. Homburger's attention. I accepted the offer and we looked forward to the challenges presented at Tufts in Boston. Dr. Welch told me he expected me to calm Freddie down. I was soon to find out what he meant— this expectation turned out to be most difficult to achieve. The change from Chicago to Boston became a most significant milestone.

CHAPTER 10

BOSTON AND TUFTS UNIVERSITY SCHOOL OF MEDICINE

I was the lead scout in arranging our move to Boston. While my family remained in Calgary with Lil's parents, I was able to secure an apartment on Beacon Street in Boston's Back Bay district. It was the entire second floor of a classic town house with huge windows and several fireplaces. It represented a real improvement in our living conditions and I was so anxious to receive the family at South station and to escort them to our Boston residence. Not to be!

Lil and the two children arrived on the Chicago train but detrained at Back Bay Station. In the meanwhile, I was in South Station becoming more frantic by the minute as they were not among the passengers, nor were they still on the train. Finally, I telephoned my office and learned that my family had taken a taxi to our Beacon Street home. I found the three of them on the doorstep demanding an explanation of why I did not meet them at the station. All I could do was to present my bouquet of flowers and shake my head silently.

This shaky beginning was followed by the excitement of falling in love with Boston and getting settled into what appeared to be a challenging and rosy future. We were befriended by David Geller who was a former Winnipeg native and then was in the public relations business. He was also active with Tufts University and gave me some guidance into the workings of that institution.

Freddy Homburger was a dynamic, ambitious individual, about 6 feet and 2 inches tall, 220 pounds who enjoyed a bohemian iconoclastic view of life which he could afford from a financially secure base. His charming wife, Gin, was reputed to be one of the heir's of the Swiss Nestle company. She was swept off her feet in medical school by the ardent Freddy Homburger. They purchased an old large colonial home in Dedham and immediately cut out a niche for themselves in Boston society particularly in the art world.

The naive Fishmans found themselves bedazzled by the Homburgers. Parties at their home started at 6 in the evening with dinner being served at 9 P.M. The three hours in between were filled with martinis, bourbon and scotch drinks without end. As we staggered through the buffet line, we began to see that life in Boston was to be a whole lot different than it was in Chicago.

For us, an exciting event was the purchase of our first automobile—a Studebaker. I had graduated from Driver's School, had passed the Massachusetts Division of Motor Vehicles driving test and now could join mainstream America. The car was essential for my role as the Scientific Director of the Tufts Cancer Research and Cancer Control Unit. Our headquarters were located in 2,000 sq. ft. of laboratory and office space in the Ziskind building of the New England Center Hospital. However, the Unit operated a laboratory service at the Jewish Memorial Hospital in Roxbury and at the Holy Ghost Hospital in Cambridge. I supervised clinical research laboratories at these three hospitals and participated in medical rounds as well. The latter two hospitals were populated mainly by patients with chronic or terminal disease.

Aside from my commitments to clinical trials and to tumor marker studies, I was expected to compete for grants from the National Cancer Institute to support my own research. I also held a joint research professorship in the biochemistry department. It was in serious decline. However, I succeeded in introducing into the laboratory course, those experiments from which the medical students at Bowman-Gray had benefitted the most. Dr. Halvor Christenson had just become the Chairman after his stay at

Children's Hospital in Boston. He welcomed my participation at first but as the years went by, my role was gradually reduced to one lecture a year. I was to have this experience repeated once more in the biochemistry department when Dr. Alton Meister succeeded Christenson, and again later in the Pathology department under Dr. Martin Flax. It was much later that I realized that "teaching hours" were credentials to the award of tenure.

GRADUATE AND OTHER STUDENTS

One of the attractions of my joint appointment, I thought, was the opportunity to supervise the thesis work of Ph.D. graduate students along the lines of my own experiences as a graduate student in Toronto. In all my twenty-eight years at Tufts not a single Tufts graduate student was assigned to me by the Chairman of the biochemistry department. It seems that although there were far more qualified candidates than slots for thesis supervision the policy was to exclude Fishman from the graduate program.

That I was qualified, was proven by a student, Olive Pettingill, from Boston University's Department of Biology who successfully completed her Ph.D. thesis and published two papers, one (17) in the *Journal of Biological Research* and one in *Experimental Cell Research* (18). The only reason which became more and more credible to me was that Fishman was regarded as competition and the departmental power structure saw no advantage in routing graduate students my way.

However, I became a mentor to two categories of undergraduate students who were interested in biochemical cancer research. One was a large number of Tufts' undergraduate students and students from other universities who applied on their own and worked in the summer break. The other was an equal number who were members of Northeastern University's work-study program. Altogether their names appeared as co-authors on 41 papers.

The control of American postdoctoral students was in the hands of the Chairmen of the University biochemistry departments from 1948 to at least 1970. The leading departments all had funds from NIH for graduate and postgraduate training. The new Ph.D. graduates would be shuttled for postdoctoral study from one such university department to another university - in other words a type of cartel. How was a maverick scientist to find postdoctoral students?

The value of the post-doctoral students to the professor is that they brought with them the expertise and thinking of the laboratories from which they originated. In addition, their careers were dependent on the success of their post-doctoral training... hence, strong motivation.

MY FIRST JAPANESE POSTDOCTORAL STUDENT

In the late 1950s, the opportunity to receive post-doctoral training in the United States was most attractive to Japanese.

A Dr. Masao Wakabayashi from Kobe, Japan, applied for a position for postdoctoral training. At that time he was required to obtain a medical clearance from the U.S. Army Corps in Japan. After I accepted him and he was in the last weeks of preparing to come, he failed the medical examination because of a spot on his lung x-ray film. He wrote that I should not be obligated to take him. One year later he was cleared for an Exchange Visitor Visa and, of course, I accepted him.

He and his wife arrived in Boston in the fall of 1958. They were a handsome couple and we became good friends. His industry and commitment led after 18 months to the publication of three papers on ß-glucuronidase.

At this particular time, a firm in Illinois headed by Ezra Levin was preparing dehydrated defatted bovine tissue products. He was interested to find out if these organ powders retained enzyme activity. They were rich in ß-glucuronidase activity. He listed these materials in his catalogue and expressed the activity in "Fishman" units. To this day, the Sigma catalogue expresses a number of ß-glucuronidase preparations in Fishman units.

One time in November, 1959, Wakabayashi asked me if I would consider accepting an invitation to be the keynote speaker in Japan at a Symposium on Glucuronic Acid. He represented the sponsor. My response was a "yes, but"; yes I would be happy to accept, but I couldn't go without Lil. Shortly afterwards he informed me that the sponsor would agree to support the expenses for the two of us. How did this happen?

It appears that Professor Morizo Ishidate, Dean of the Faculty of Pharmaceutical Sciences at the University of Tokyo was very interested in ß-glucuronidase and glucuronic acid metabolism. He had synthesized glucuronolactone which is an inhibitor of ß-glucuronidase and had transferred his technology to the Chugai Pharmaceutical Company. They made an "across-the-counter" alka-seltzer-like product "guronsan" which was very popular with the public. Every year, a symposium on glucuronic acid was held and I was invited to the Fifth Glucuronic Acid Symposium, the first Westerner honored in this way.

The invitation that Masao Wakabayashi brought from Dr. Ishidate made it possible for the Fishman family to enjoy a unique experience. The six weeks we spent in Japan in the summer of 1959 became a major turning point and milestone in our lives and in the future success of the scientific program.

A Pan-American four propeller engine plane bore us from the West Coast to Wake Island where we landed in the middle of the night for a refueling stop. We landed in late morning at Haneda airport. Two uniformed men entered the plane and asked for Dr. Fishman to identify himself. After our family stood up we were escorted out of the plane. On the tarmac awaiting to greet us were

Dr. and Mrs. Morizo Ishidate. She presented Lil with a huge bouquet of flowers while the cameras rolled. Dr. Ishidate was a tall handsome man who radiated pleasure on seeing us. When we prepared to go through immigration and customs, he asked for our passports and baggage stubs which he turned over to several of the uniformed personnel. It turned out they were graduates of his faculty at the University of Tokyo. We sailed through like royalty! The Fishman family were placed in two limousines and altogether our entourage consisted of four limousines wending their way through Tokyo's narrow streets.

We arrived at Frank Lloyd Wright's Imperial Hotel, the one that had survived Tokyo's most devastating earthquake. A spacious suite was assigned to us and we had several hours of free time. Then there was a knock at the door. It was a Chugai representative who gave us two detailed schedules; one for Dr. Fishman's lectures and visits to institutions, the other for Lil, Joel, Nina and Daniel for their rounds of entertainment. The knock at the door was to occur frequently and on time as listed in the itineraries. The youngsters would regularly exclaim, "the Chugai's are here" in response to the knock on the door.

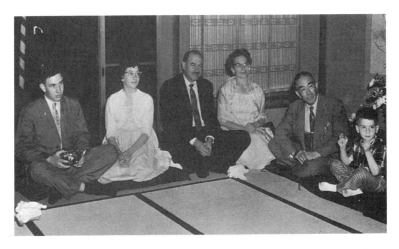

Entertainment at the home of Juzo Uyeno, Founder of the Chugai Pharmaceutical Co.
l. to r.: Joel, Nina, Bill, Lil, Mr. Oda, Daniel - 1959

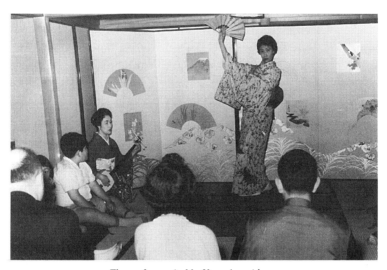

The performer in Mr. Uyena's residence

There was no accommodation for jet lag in those days. On the first evening we were chauffeured to the estate of the president of the Chugai Pharmaceutical Company, Mr. Juzo Uyeno. We were greeted warmly, Japanese style, with the whole household lined up to greet us, and escorted to the site of the garden party located in the midst of a formal Japanese garden. Juzo Uyeno was a powerfully-built man who projected warmth, understanding, and leadership. He donned the chef's apron with a big smile and personally served us various delicacies. Standing behind us were beautiful ladies in obi and kimono who kept our glasses for sake and beer filled at all times. Dr. and Mrs. Morizo Ishidate were seated with us.

After dinner we were ushered into a large room where we were seated on tatami grass mats. We were then entertained by classic Geisha dancers performing to the music of the Samesan and Kota stringed instruments. There, we experienced the beauty of Japanese culture for the first time.

We were then ushered in to a Western Parlor where we could sit on chairs. There, very ceremoniously, gifts were presented to the family (one had to remove the wrappings carefully for fear of tearing the elegant handmade paper)— a camera for Joel, jewelry for Lil and Nina and a transistor radio for Daniel. Accustomed as we were to a spartan routine in Boston, our introduction to traditional Japanese hospitality almost turned our heads.

For the next six weeks the Fishman family toured Japan as guests of the Chugai pharmaceutical company. I delivered lectures to the Japanese Cancer Society, Japanese Biochemical Society and the Japanese Pharmaceutical Society after the conclusion of the Fifth Glucuronic Acid Symposium. The academic institutions at which I gave addresses included the Universities of Tokyo, Nagoya, Gifu, Kyoto, and Kyushu;. At each of these, my host was a colleague or former student of Dr. Ishidate with the Chugai representative taking care of all the hotel and travel arrangements.

The typical visit and lecture can be described as follows. First, I would meet with the Professor in his sitting room - and everyone was served a cup of green tea. My lantern slides, two sets to be shown simultaneously on two screens, were taken to the projectionist. I was then introduced to my interpreter, who was usually someone from the humanities faculty or the customs department. These individuals had the greatest difficulty understanding me and my subject so a great deal was "lost in the translation." My talk was an hour in length, the translation was also an hour and this was not the end of it. We all then moved to another smaller lecture hall where faculty and graduate students questioned me. But this time the room for error was magnified. The interpreter had to translate the questions from Japanese to English, I answered what I thought the question was and my answer was translated back into Japanese by an interpreter who I believed understood very imperfectly both the question and the answer. This took another two hours. I found this exercise demanding on both my mental and physical capacities. The social exercises were strenuous also, with each visit including a reception and a dinner at which formal greetings, toasts, and speeches were exchanged.

The typical day for my family was very educational. They were taken to silk factories, pottery and china museums, temples, shrines, and Japanese theatre. We had a lot to report to each other every night.

There were some interludes which were most refreshing and interesting. One was a visit to Hakone hot springs not far from Tokyo. We were assigned a cottage under which a small stream flowed...the sound of the water was very calming. The Ishidates took us to one locality after another to try to catch a glimplse of Mount Fuji. To their and our disappointment, Mt Fuji remained invisible under cloud cover. Another was the evening at Gifu when we embarked on boats to observe the cormorant fishermen maneuver their birds to fish for the small trout "ayu". A ring on the bird's neck prevented the passage of the fish into their gullets. The birds obligingly disgorged their catch when they were returned to the boat. A dinner of baked "ayu" was served by kimono-clad ladies who also kept filling our sake and beer glasses. Finally, there was the trip from Fukuoka to Kumamoto where we visited a live volcano. It was an awesome experience as we ascended to the rim of its crater to view the desolate landscape in which fire and smoke escaped from cracks and fissures in the black lava. It was as good a picture of hell as one could imagine. On this trip I met Dr. Tadeo Takeuchi and his wife who became our very good personal and professional friends.

We scheduled a stop in Honolulu on our way back to Boston. The tranquility of the beach, the warm winds of the Pacific, the return to a western style all combined to completely rest my brain and body. So much so that we checked out of the hotel, went to the airport only to find that the Canadian Pacific plane left Honolulu the next day. I had forgotten to adjust to our eastern passage over the international dateline. To my chagrin we returned to Honolulu and with luck secured lodging for the night. We made it back to Boston without further incident.

Our experiences in Japan had made a profound difference in our lives. It expanded our horizons, introduced us to a completely different culture and resulted in our making life-long friendships.

Masao Wakabayashi was the first of nearly twenty-five Japanese postdoctoral students who worked with me in Boston and in La Jolla. All these visiting students did well, worked hard and intelligently, and were co-authors on many papers in first-class journals. One is now a Dean of Pharmaceutical Sciences in Kyushu University, some are chairmen and professors of departments of pathology, obstetrics and gynecology, and biochemistry and others have advanced into management positions in industry.

Three success stories of undergraduate medical students who had their first laboratory experiences with me merit description.

Leo L. Stolbach was an undergraduate at Harvard and completed his M.D. at the University of Rochester. In the summers he learned how to conduct assay procedures for acid phosphatase and its L-tartrate-sensitive isozyme of prostatic origin. This work was an extension of the discovery of Florence Lerner and myself that cancer of the prostate could be correlated best with this acid phosphatase isozyme. Leo not only became proficient in the analyses but brought a curiosity and enthusiasm to bear on the problem which was contagious. He went on to the National Cancer Institute to work with endocrinologist Roy Hertz who with M. C. Li had introduced the highly successful methotrexate chemotherapy for choriocarcinoma (19). Eventually he returned to Tufts as an oncologist and worked at the Lemuel Shattuck Hospital which had a population of chronically-ill patients many of whom were afflicted with cancer. He turned out to be the key oncologist (20) in the discovery of the Regan Isoenzyme in 1968. He is now a Professor of Medicine at the University of

Massachusetts Medical School.

Ronald DeLellis, first came to the laboratory as a sophomore medical student. He combined his talent for histology and cytology with histochemistry in a whole range of investigations and published his findings on the dual localization of ß-glucuronidase in lysosomes and in endoplasmic reticulum. This study appeared in *Nature* as a lead article (21). It was a major contribution. He also did his post-doctoral work at the National Cancer Institute working for Dr. George Glenner. Glenner later demonstrated ß-amyloid in the brains of patients with Alzheimers disease. Today, DeLellis is a Professor of Pathology at Tufts and a leading scholar in histochemistry. His book on immunohistopathology is a classic.

Phillip Fialkow, an undergraduate medical student, came to the laboratory to work with me on ß-glucuronidase. He produced an original paper (22) published in the *Journal of Biological Chemistry* and impressed me with the depth of his scholarship. As a faculty member of the University of Washington he pioneered in collecting experimental evidence supporting the clonal origin of cancer using isozyme markers. Today he is the Dean of the School of Medicine at the University of Washington. My laboratory was the source of a number of weddings and Phil's was the first. Helen Dimitrakis, an expert technician in the histochemistry lab, won Phil's heart. They were married the summer he graduated and moved to San Francisco for his residency.

CHAPTER 11

ORIGINS OF THE TUFTS CANCER RESEARCH CENTER

In 1948, with his experiences at Sloan-Kettering Memorial Hospital in the clinical investigation of cancer still fresh, Freddy Homburger poured his energy and intellect into building a Cancer Research and Cancer Control Unit in the Department of Surgery. He regarded the existing Faculty and administration as mediocre and made the mistake of communicating these opinions all the way up to the President of the University.

Some of the lessons he learned at the New York institution were ill-suited for a small New England college. He believed that you have "to break the eggs in order to make an omelette." Consequently, he rode roughshod over the feelings of his colleagues in his hurry to achieve immediate success.

Nevertheless, the Cancer Research and Cancer Control Unit of which I was the Associate Director rapidly assumed a leadership role in challenging the medical students and residents to address cancer as a subject requiring study throughout the medical school curriculum and beyond. Oncology rounds were instituted at the bedside of cancer patients at the Jewish Memorial Hospital in Roxbury and the Holy Ghost Hospital in Cambridge. New chemotherapeutic drugs were introduced. This was the age of Sidney Farber's success with methotrexate in treating leukemia, of David Karnovsky's use of alkylating agents and of Herz and Li's management of choriocarcinoma with methotrexate. For me, this was a "hands-on" educational experience in which I learned of the problems which confronted the clinical oncologist. It became clear that "palliation" was important to achieve first and that remission and cure were very distant.

My role was to define a clinical problem that one might hope to solve by a laboratory procedure. My preference was for an enzyme test. The measurement of acid phosphatase in the serum of patients with prostatic cancer had been found to be useful in the differential diagnosis of the disease and in its management. However, the test was relatively insensitive and produced false positives if the serum samples were contaminated with even a trace of hemolyzed erythrocytes. (Erythrocytes are rich in acid phosphatase.) Early in 1949, several British workers (23) reported that one could distinguish prostatic and erythrocytic acid phosphatase with the inhibitor, L-tartrate. We succeeded in developing an assay (24) for "prostatic" acid phosphatase in serum which avoided the many false positives. It was more specific than the existing techniques for prostatic cancer. The consequence of this research was the acceptance by urologic oncologists of the new technique and its value in making the differential diagnosis of prostatic cancer. The test was used widely in teaching hospitals associated with medical schools. In the 1970s it was superseded by radioimmunoassay technology and in the 1990s by the PSA method.

The National Cancer Institute in 1950 set up several programs for the evaluation of tumor markers. The field was inundated with empirical cancer tests which lacked a relevant rationale. There was the Penn Test which interpreted the microscopic pattern of a dried mixture of a drop of the patients' blood with a reagent derived from human tissues; also being promoted was the Huggins-Jensen test which alleged the lack of coagulability of the serum of cancer patients, and many others. Our outfit was one of the NCI Centers, and my laboratory did the evaluations on blood specimens provided by the clinical oncologists. Thus, began my education in critically evaluating cancer tests.

ACTH AND THE ARTIST, RAOUL DUFY

In 1950, the Armour Company in Chicago had succeeded in preparing substantial amounts of ACTH from bovine pituitary glands. This product was in great demand after Dr. Phillip Hench at Mayo's had demonstrated its effectiveness in correcting the handicaps of arthritic patients. Dr. Mote, Armour's clinical director, arranged a Symposium to collect the new information and to make ACTH available to clinical research groups. Freddy Homburger and I attended.

Although Freddy was able to benefit a variety of patients with ACTH he will be remembered best for his treatment of his most famous patient, the French impressionist artist, Raoul Dufy. Dufy was suffering from crippling osteoarthritis which prevented him from painting. Freddy contacted Dufy and arranged a bed for him at the Jewish Memorial Hospital. Imagine the excitement when Dufy arrived with his entourage and settled into a stay of several months. The ACTH worked and Dufy was able to paint again in his colorful style. Although I was the key to the laboratory studies, it turned out that only the clinicians received paintings from Dufy. However, when Gene Roberts and I visited him in his Paris studio several years later in 1952 he very graciously presented each of us with a poster which he autographed.

WHAT ABOUT MY RESEARCH DIRECTION?

It seemed important to me to lose no time in exploring the possible clinical benefit of our laboratory findings. The most promising lead was to compare the performance of the PAP smear test for cervical cancer with vaginal fluid ß-glucuronidase. This lead originated from our Chicago studies in which we found high concentrations of ß-glucuronidase in cancer of the uterine cervix and other organs. Thus, it was reasonable to expect that the enzyme would enrich the vaginal fluid.

Accordingly, Dr. S. Charles Kasdon, of the Department of Obstetrics and Gynecology and I organized a lab-clinical study which culminated in publications (25,26) in the *Journal of the American Medical Association*. Although a positive correlation was established, the PAP smear remained the more feasible one for the medical practitioner.

By 1950, the National Cancer Institute was becoming a major source of research funds which were awarded on a competitive basis. The investigator submitted an R01-application in which specific aims were defined, an experimental plan to accomplish these aims, a review of the investigator's contributions to the field, and a budget. The application was routed to an appropriate Study Section. A Study Section consisted of between twelve to sixteen scientists appointed on the basis of relevant expertise, geography, race, and gender. Meeting three times a year, the Study Section evaluated about one hundred applications at each meeting and ranked them in order of merit. The applications would be funded from the highest rank down until all the research money had been committed.

In 1947, I was successful in receiving an NCI award to investigate the hormonal induction of ß-glucuronidase in mouse uterus. Support of this study and its many interesting extensions was awarded to me competitively for the next thirty years.

The isozyme nature of the L-tartrate-sensitive acid phosphatase was the basis of another NCI Grant which continued for over two decades.

In 1956, I began to study the isozymes of alkaline phosphatase in relation to disease including cancer. This research continued until 1989, competing successfully for NIH funds during this period.

In order to win "investigator-initiated" (R01) grants and still maintain my reputation as a basic scientist it was necessary for me to travel on two tracks. One was the basic science track of accomplishment documented by publication in prestigious journals such as *Nature, Journal of Biological Chemistry, Endocrinology*, and *Journal of Histochemistry and Cytochemistry.* The other track was in oncology and in laboratory-clinical investigations which were supported by institutional grants and the results were published in the *New England Journal of Medicine, Cancer Research*, etc. For a very long time, scientists who were committed to cancer research were regarded as second-class by the biochemistry establishment and accordingly it was necessary for cancer researchers to renew their biochemical credentials periodically in order to compete.

The publication of Hoeber's Homburger-Fishman treatise on the *Physiopathology of Cancer* in 1953 was widely read and appreciated. Later, Academic Press published my three-volume treatise on Metabo*lic Hydrolysis and Metabolic Conjugation*, Volume 18 of Methods in Cancer Research entitled *Oncodevelopmental Antigens* in 1979 and *Oncodevelopmental Markers; Biologic, Diagnostic and Monitoring Effects*, 1983. My monograph on *Drug Metabolism* was published by Wiley and Co.

EXIT FREDDY HOMBURGER

Freddy imagined himself as another Cornelius "Dusty" Rhoads—he was the one who had developed the Sloan-Kettering Institute into a major cancer research center. "Dusty" Rhoads was a master politician in attracting huge grants from the National Cancer Institute, building a brilliant staff of scientists and clinicians and forming successful strategic alliances with figures such as Mary Lasker and Sidney Farber. The medical school of Tufts College lacked financial and physical resources necessary for the efforts of a second "Dusty" Rhoads. From a personality point of view there developed a hostility between Freddy and both the Medical School Dean and the President of the University. This was believed by Dr. K. Dobriner of the Sloan-Kettering Institute, to be a consequence of Freddy's inappropriate use of American expletives to publicly describe these officers of the University.

In 1955, Freddy had decided that he did not see his future continuing at Tufts and so he looked for and found what seemed to be a better opportunity. It appeared that Dr. Sidney Farber at the Cancer Center of the Childrens Hospital had an option to space and oncology services in an adjacent hospital. Freddy planned to move the entire Cancer Research and Cancer Control Unit from Tufts to Harvard. In the process, however, he promoted Dr. Peter Bernfeld, to the same rank I held in the Unit.

Dr. Bernfeld was a European biochemist with whom Freddy felt more comfortable than he did with me, probably because they both shared a Swiss background. Bernfeld was supported in large part by my grants on ß-glucuronidase and the two of us along with Jerry Nisselbaum published good papers (27,28) in the Journal of *Biological Chemistry*.

A MAJOR DECISION

For several weeks, I wrestled with a decision which would affect my career and family for the rest of my life. My research studies were going well, being funded by ROI-grants from the National Cancer Institute—my staff was experienced and enthusiastic—my salary was provided from the Cancer Teaching grant—my relationship with my colleagues and the Administration were proper and cordial. I did not have such an appetite for a Harvard appointment that nothing else mattered.

It also became clear that Freddy and Peter were excluding

me from their planning and discussions—suggesting that my future role was to undergo a change for the worse not the better.

In Freddy's maneuvering at Tufts in 1956, it was clear he was using me and the research program as a shield to power his agenda at Tufts. Also, I resented having myself and my career being used as a political tool in his personal battles with the Dean and the President. My destiny was in his hands.

Lil and I discussed the pros and cons of the decision at great length finally agreeing to stay at Tufts and not to move to Harvard. I notified Freddy of this decision in a long letter and then made clear to the Tufts Administration my continuing loyalty to the University and my intention to stay.

There was a cost to this decision. In the eyes of the research community the names of Homburger and Fishman constituted one identity. When these names were separated in 1956, the majority opinion was that Homburger, the M.D., was the one who secured the funding and directed the research program. Fishman, the Ph.D., was a relatively unknown quantity except for his research publications. Would the granting agencies accept Fishman as Homburger's successor at Tufts? Would the opposition which Freddy generated be visited on Fishman? Did Fishman have the administrative ability to manage the Cancer Research and Cancer Control Unit? How vindictive would Freddy be?

After Freddy resigned at Tufts, he encountered a major reverse. Dr. Farber and he had a disagreement and the move to Harvard was called off. This created a tense situation. Tufts University was happy to have Freddy terminate his appointment and was firmly opposed to his recovering his position. In the laboratory, relations between our two staffs became strained. My position was changed to Acting Director by Tufts and so had the responsibility of managing the fortunes and misfortunes of the organization. This was a turbulent period and I became the target of Homburger's hostility.

How was this impasse resolved? Freddy discussed his career problems with Dr. Shields Warren, formerly head of the Medical Division of the Atomic Energy Commission. Warren proposed that since Freddy was a free spirit, he establish his own enterprise independent of academia. This was the answer to Freddy's problems. In just a few weeks he created the Bioresearch Institute in Cambridge and Peter Bernfeld, John Baker and others joined him and he transferred his grants to that organization.

I felt liberated! The control of the laboratory, its research program and its future direction were now my responsibility and I could compete for grant funds to support them. If I failed it was not due to the machinations of my chief and if I succeeded, it was due to merit alone. In time the scientific community would have sufficient evidence to judge the degree of accomplishment merited by each of the Homburger-Fishman names.

The key to survival by faculty members who were not tenured was their ability to compete successfully for research grants from the National Institutes of Health and the American Cancer Society. In the 1950s and 1960s non-tenured faculty were completely out of the power structure of the Institution and received little or no "hard" money from their departments. "Hard" money was the University's revenue derived from student fees and income on investments and was controlled by the Dean and the Department Chairmen.

TEACHING EXPERIENCES AT TUFTS

The biochemistry department chairman from 1955 to 1967 was Dr. Alton Meister. His interest was centered on amino acid metabolism and the advancement of his career. He succeeded Dr. Halvor Christensen who had supervised the move of the Department from its Huntington Avenue location to its present site on Harrison Avenue. His acceptance of an appointment at the

University of Michigan created the vacancy Meister was to fill.

Although I was acquainted with Meister from his days at the National Cancer Institute and offered him my cooperation, he identified me immediately as a competitor. He once said "you guys trap a lot of money over there." I sought to have the adjective "research" removed from the title of professor in view of the considerable amount of teaching I and others in the "soft" money positions did. This produced an emotional reaction from Meister which surprised me and resulted in his cancelling my teaching responsibilities. From then on, our relationship became cool and distant. Applications of graduate students or postdoctoral students never were routed my way.

During this interval, Dr. Ed MacMahon, the chairman of the Pathology Department wanted to have basic research going on in his arena. There was little or none at the time. He invited me to join his department and to deliver six lectures on the "Biology of Cancer" to the medical students. I accepted and my title became "Research Professor of Pathology (Oncology)."

EARLY EFFORTS IN LABORATORY/CLINICAL RESEARCH

The National Cancer Institute had organized several major initiatives which involved the participation of medical schools. One was the search for drugs with chemotherapeutic potential and another was clinical trials to evaluate the safety and efficacy of the promising candidate drugs. Still another was to support radiology cancer centers inasmuch as the U.S. was far behind Sweden which was having success in treating cancer with radiation.

At Tufts, the medical oncology group was headed by Dr. Mel Krant, oncology chief at the State's Lemuel Shattuck Hospital and his colleagues, Drs. Joseph Cohen and Leo L. Stolbach. Leo, my summer research assistant, had worked in endocrinologic oncology with Dr. Roy Hertz at the National Cancer Institute for three years prior to returning to Boston. The Shattuck Hospital was a chronic disease hospital with over one hundred cancer patients receiving therapy.

At the New England Center Hospital, Dr. Larry Nathanson ran the medical oncology service dealing mainly with short-term management of recently diagnosed cancer patients.

In a very short time, active cooperative studies were initiated by the Fishman laboratory and the Medical Oncology group which centered on isozyme studies. These were highly productive and established the credibility of an operational lab-clinical program.

Also at the New England Center Hospital, Dr. Fernando Bloedorn established a Radiology Cancer Center equipped with the state of the art cobalt machines. He supported a radiology biology laboratory headed by Dr. Donald Wallach.

In the 1960s the National Cancer Institute recognized multidisciplinary cancer centers to which they awarded block grants e.g. Sloan-Kettering Memorial Hospital, New York and the M.D. Anderson Cancer Hospital, Houston. By the time President Richard Nixon signed the National "war on cancer" Act in 1972, the concept had found wide-spread support for the creation of a number of cancer centers, both basic and clinical, across the nation. An Institution, in order to compete, had to apply for a "planning" grant which would provide short-term support for it to organize a Center "Core" Grant application. Tufts prepared a planning grant under Mel Krant's supervision. Trouble began as soon as the award was made because of a power struggle between the Lemuel Shattuck Hospital group, the New England Center Hospital's Medical Oncology and Radiology Oncology group, the surgeons and the Medical School Dean. My perception was that there was economic benefit to whichever group took possession of the Center—medical oncologists, radiologists, surgeons,—and not one of these disciplines would recognize the relevance of the other.

Finally, Dean W. C. Maloney; appointed me to replace Krant as the Principal Investigator of the Planning Grant. I, as a Ph.D. earning no patient fees, was not a threat to the clinicians, was widely recognized, and besides I was highly regarded by the NCI as an original cancer researcher.

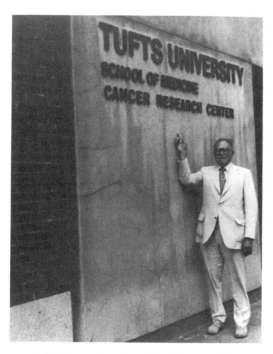

Bill Fishman, Founder and first Director of the
Tufts University Cancer Research Center, 1975

HISTORY OF THE DISCOVERY OF THE REGAN ISOENZYME; THE PLAP TUMOR MARKER

In 1953, my laboratory had devised a specific method for measuring the acid phosphatase of prostatic origin. This isoenzyme was inhibited by L-tartrate. It was evaluated by Dr. Wyland Ledbetter of the Urology department of the Massachusetts

General Hospital. He observed that in the presence of digital evidence of a prostate lesion, a positive test indicated spread of the disease beyond the prostate capsule (29). Hormonal therapy only was the recommended therapy. On the other hand, if under these circumstances the test was negative, then radical prostatectomy was the treatment of choice. The so-called Fishman-Lerner method was highly regarded by urologists and oncologists in helping to solve problems in differential diagnosis.

After I had delivered a seminar on the application of enzymology to clinical oncology at the Montefiore hospital in New York, I was engaged in conversation with Dr. Daniel Lazlo, then Chief of Clinical Oncology. He implored me to tackle a problem which was bedevilling the staff. He described the difficulty of interpreting the significance of an elevation of serum alkaline phosphatase in metastatic breast cancer in response to chemotherapy. The elevation could be interpreted in two ways; one—that healing of bone by alkaline phosphatase-rich osteoblasts was taking place; or the other that an exacerbation of hepatic metastases occured. It was clearly important to produce methods which could distinguish between liver and bone alkaline phosphatase.

Here then was a clinical oncologist who defined a real need which an enzymologist could be expected to tackle. I accepted the challenge.

Since isozyme-specific inhibitors, e.g. L-tartrate inhibitable acid phosphatase, had worked so well in the differential diagnosis of prostatic cancer, I initiated a systematic study of every compound which had been reported to inhibit alkaline phosphatase. The purpose was to determine if any of them had organ specificity. The organs included liver, bone, spleen, kidney, intestine and serum. We did find organ specificity but not of the type we were searching for.

Thus, L-phenylalanine inhibited intestinal alkaline phosphatase unlike D-phenylalanine under the same conditions (30). L-homoarginine inhibited the liver isozyme but not the intestine or bone isozymes. The work of others had demonstrated that the bone alkaline phosphatase was especially sensitive to heat treatment. With the help of Sid Green and Norma Inglis an automated technicon method (31) was devised which ultimately yielded a fractionation of the liver, bone and intestinal alkaline phosphatases. The same inhibitors and heat inactivation were subsequently employed to identify individual isozyme bands in electrophoretic gels.

One isozyme which attracted our interest was of placental origin. It had been recognized (32) as an enzyme which could survive exposure to 100°C and was first found as a contaminant of placental albumin. The rise in serum alkaline phosphatase which followed the injection of placental albumin alarmed clinicians but the patients had no liver or bone disorders. The alarm abated when the nature of the contaminant was established as placental alkaline phosphatase (32).

We engaged in a systematic study of this unique placental alkaline phosphatase including its complete purification, its enzyme kinetics and its exponential increase during the second and third trimester of pregnancy.

It was a fortunate circumstance that Leo L. Stolbach had joined the oncology staff of the Tufts service at the Lemuel Shattuck hospital in suburban Boston. Together we decided to fractionate the serum alkaline phosphatase isozymes in the blood of cancer and non-cancer patients.

The study yielded a wealth of information which enabled us to correctly interpret the significance of the elevation of alkaline phosphatase values in metastatic breast cancer patients receiving chemotherapy.

DISCOVERY OF THE REGAN ISOENZYME - PLAP

However, the most interesting result was the behavior of the isozymes in the serum of a patient, Peter Regan, with metastatic lung cancer. This was a thirty-two year-old teacher who smoked two to three packs of cigarettes a day over the years. What arrested our attention was the fact that most of his alkaline phosphatase was completely heat-stable. When the analysis was repeated a week later, the amount of this heat-stable alkaline phosphatase had doubled. It was most important to determine whether this was the placental isozyme.

Electrophoretically, it was quickly observed that the isozyme migrated to the placental position. The problem had by now defined itself—was the isozyme in Peter Regan's blood placental alkaline phosphatase—(PLAP)? One feasible approach was to test the isozyme with specific rabbit antisera to PLAP with Cinader's antigen-retardation electrophoretic technique. The answer—Regan's isozyme was PLAP.

Although the circulation was enriched with PLAP what was the tissue of origin? This could only be answered by a study of the patient's tissues. We did not have long to wait. He was admitted as an emergency to the St. Elizabeth's hospital and died a couple of days later. A Tufts senior medical student on rotation had become aware of the interest at the Shattuck hospital in Mr. Regan's isozyme of alkaline phosphatase during rounds with Dr. Stolbach. He then sought and received authorization to secure a variety of benign and malignant tissue samples at autopsy. These were then delivered to the Fishman laboratory.

We were able to demonstrate that all the enzymic kinetics, immunologic and physical properties of Regan's isozyme were indistinguishable from authentic PLAP. Also, by the use of specific enzyme histochemical methods, it was unequivocally proven that this isozyme was generated in the cancer cells, exclusively. All the members of the Fishman lab and the Stolbach clinic were thrilled and excited with this striking result (33).

For days I was asking myself this question. What is a man with terminal lung cancer doing making a placental protein in such abundance? The next question which preoccupied me was— what was the significance of a tumor producing an extraembryonic membrane protein? It was these two questions which gave rise to my oncodevelopmental view of cancer.

With the help of Leo Stolbach and Larry Nathanson (34) it was possible to evaluate the presence of PLAP in a variety of human cancers (20,33). The most frequent occurrence in order was testis, ovary and pancreas. The serum level correlated with events of regression and recurrence during long-term longitudinal studies of cancer patients. Today, the work of Millán, Stigbrand and Lange (35) have focussed on seminoma which has been proven to produce a germ cell alkaline phosphatase which has been referred in the earlier literature as "placental-like". Also, Epenetos (36) and his colleagues in London using PLAP antibodies, have successfully applied radioimmunolocalization and radioimmunotherapy to patients with ovarian and other malignancies.

At the time of the discovery of the Regan isozyme. I learned of two observations which appeared relevant to the question of the basic significance of our work. One was the independent reports of Abelev (37) and Tatarinov (38) of the re-expression in mouse and human liver cancer (hepatomas) of an embryonic yolk sac and liver alpha-fetoprotein (AFP). The other was reported in a paper by Gold and Freeman (39) that human colon cancers expressed an antigen which matched a fetal intestinal antigen. It was termed "carcinoembryonic antigen," CEA.

In experimental tumors in rats, Schapira (40) and Weinhouse (41) had earlier demonstrated the strong expression of the fetal forms of the key enzymes of the respiratory chain. This explained the propensity of tumors to undergo anaerobic glycolysis, a phenomenon that Otto Warburg had studied.

However, trophoblastic proteins had a different biological niche than liver or colon tissue proteins or the respiratory cycle component enzymes. These specialized trophoblast proteins at the time of implantation of the fertilized egg participated in invasive phenomena and rapid multiplication which had their counterparts in cancer cells. The idea that aberrant rests of trophoblastic cells gave rise to cancer in the adult had been advanced by Beard in 1901.

It was not essential to prove that individually AFP, CEA, or PLAP were gene products that were either important in the etiology of cancer or were the consequences of the neoplastic event. What was important was that oncology was inextricably a manifestation of developmental biology and that to understand the role of an embryonic gene product in the tumor it is essential to know its role in the particular developmental phase in which it is normally expressed. Many years later, some of the embryonic gene products or their mutated forms have been identified as oncogenes and as tumor suppressor genes. The specific embryonic gene is termed a protooncogene. Finally all of the key initial phenomena are taking place in the DNA of specific chromosomes in the nucleus of living cells. Thus it is the DNA which is the site of damage produced by chemical carcinogens, radiation and genetic mutations. This event, termed initiation, when followed by an interval of exposure to agents which promote cell division leads eventually to cancer.

THE TUFTS CANCER RESEARCH CENTER IS BORN

Taking on the responsibility of organizing a cancer center was a major milestone in my career. I was attracted by the first sentence of the NCI guidelines which stated that "the Cancer

Center must have a scientific mission." If, as the Principal Investigator, I could fashion the scientific mission as one towards which I and other Tufts faculty could pool our efforts, then it all would be worthwhile. This mission was articulated as the "oncodevelopmental concept" which will be discussed in detail later.

I recall innumerable meetings and crises. One powerful hematologic oncologist stated "Fishman, this grant represents a sack of money and each of us has a right to reach in and to take what we need." My strategy then was to include every project which was submitted by the faculty and let the NCI site visit committee decide which ones merited funding. Of sixteen projects, six were approved and all of these had relevance to the oncodevelopmental concept. The hematologists' project was denied.

The Site Visit committee headed by Dr. Al Gelhorn recognized the multidisciplinary research opportunity which the grant represented and awarded some $2,000,000. Included was about $1,000,000 to create a Clinical Bed Unit and laboratory for the New England Center Hospital, to renovate the animal room facilities and to renovate a floor in the Cancer Center building. The remainder was to be given for the six research projects and the office of the Cancer Center Director.

The climate changed at Tufts with the award of the Core Grant. I found myself without a friend. From someone who was on "soft" money and therefore expendable, I had become a figure "who had more money than the Dean." Even more disturbing to powerful members of the faculty was that I had formulated an original scientific approach to a cancer center over whose destiny they had no control. This resentment found its full expression when it was time to prepare the renewal application 18 months later.

Under the leadership of Drs. Martin Flax, Robert S. Schwartz,

Moselio Schaechter et al and with the support of the Dean, I was informed that they represented the basic cancer science effort and that henceforth my role would be limited to administering the Core Grant. Funding was planned for four programs they were formulating. I could, if I wanted, contribute to one of these programs but they would decide whether or not to include my component.

I accepted gracefully as there was nothing I could do about it. The burden of preparing four programs, each with several components with the necessary documentation of curriculum vitae, reprints etc., and of editing all this material was very heavy. We completed these four programs in time, sent it with my core administration component to Washington and waited.

We did not have to wait long. The National Cancer Institute returned the application stating it was not reviewable and one major flaw was that the previous scientific strength of the funded grant (W. H. Fishman) was not represented in the renewal application.

Dean Lauro Cavazos scheduled a meeting with me and informed me of the NCI action. Clearly, the institution was in danger not only of losing a substantial amount of research funding but of suffering a humiliating loss of prestige of its new cancer research center. My suggestion was for the Dean to give me the authority to organize a single program out of the four programs by choosing those components that were most relevant to the scientific mission and to write the application. This he did. With only a few weeks to the deadline, my staff and I succeeded in putting together a cohesive and well-documented application.

Several months later, the NCI site visit team spent two days reviewing our progress and plans for the next five years. My perception was that they were impressed by the originality of the program and by the credentials of the leadership and the participating scientists. We were successful. Earlier we were also funded for an NCI Construction Grant to renovate a floor in the Cancer Center building to accommodate two virologists, S. S. Tevethia and J. M. Coffin.

The NCI report not only dealt with the enthusiastic approval of the scientific program and the clinical coordination but made some serious recommendations. The weakness that the NCI identified was the "rootlessness" of the cancer center in the administrative structure of the Medical School. They noted that the administrative unit at Tufts was the department and that Dr. Fishman and his staff should be collected into a department of oncology inasmuch as their accomplishments over the years merited this recognition.

This possibility of receiving Tufts recognition for my prodigious effort over 26 years was a pyrrhic victory for the reason that it was the key event which set in motion my departure from Tufts.

The department chairmen were alarmed and upset by the NCI recommendation. This would mean that oncology would be assigned teaching hours and would gain departmental status equivalent to theirs. As one of them bluntly told me "Listen, Fishman your department of oncology would receive "hard" money from the University. This would mean less "hard" money for us. No way will this happen." The faces of the the Dean and the Research Coordinator were grim when we met after the NCI report.

In order to route the grant funds of the renewal application out of the responsibility and control of the Director, the Dean divided the grant in two. One part was to be administered by his Research Coordinator and the second part, by the Director. However, since the Director was held accountable by the NCI for every dollar spent of the grant funds. I felt very uneasy with the Dean's action which could be viewed as inappropriate and hostile. I now faced an involuntary loss of personal integrity since

I was being used to bring in the Center funds but others would spend half of the money without being accountable to the Director.

In 1975, it was time for me to renew my NCI five-year Career Award which provided most of my salary. Since the renewal period would extend two years beyond retirement age, I asked the Dean whether the institution would accept the grant. His answer was that after age 65, my appointment would be on a year to year basis; that I could continue with my own research but that someone else would direct the cancer center.

What were the chances that the scientific mission of the Center would be pursued under other supervision? None at all. My successor had already been chosen. He was Dr. Robert S. Schwartz, hematology-oncology service head of the New England Center Hospital. Bob was an aggressive individual who planned to fashion the Center to support his research activities which were divorced from the oncodevelopmental concept. The Dean also believed that a clinician could bring in a lot more funds to the Medical School than a Ph.D.

As I evaluated these circumstances, I concluded that there was no future for the Center program or for me at Tufts. Where there is no future, it follows there is no present. Clearly, there was absolutely no way for me to win at Tufts and the oncodevelopmental research program would be adversely affected. Lil and I agreed we should relocate to a more hospitable institution where the rules governing age at retirement would be more flexible and where there was a better opportunity to contribute to the Center's scientific mission to which I was completely committed.

After 28 years at Tufts, we decided to move on.

PART II

THE LA JOLLA CANCER
RESEARCH FOUNDATION

CHAPTER 12

WHY AND HOW IT WAS STARTED

RELOCATION? WHERE? HOW? WHEN?

We agreed that our geographic preference was California based on the reasoning that if we didn't succeed at least we would end up in a warmer climate for our retirement years. In addition, we each had close family in San Francisco and Los Angeles.

Would a University Medical School or a Teaching Hospital care to recruit me? I explored five such institutions and they were not interested for several reasons. One was that they operated under strict rules that mandated retirement at age 65. Why would they make an exception for me? Another was that they were not structured to accommodate a free-standing cancer research program.

It was then that I consulted officials at the Cancer Centers Branch of the National Cancer Institute. From the government's point of view a non-profit institution or foundation with the capability of administering research grants and accounting for the funds qualified for NCI support. I searched for such foundations and found they had other priorities which represented their funding commitments. There was only one option left and that was to create a new foundation whose sole function was to support oncodevelopmental research.

WHERE SHOULD WE RELOCATE IN CALIFORNIA?

The history of the answer to this question dates back to the fall of 1972 when a meeting was held in Sapporo, Japan, by an international group whose aim was to study carcinoembryonic proteins. Under the auspices of Drs. T. Wada and H. Hirai, a number of active researchers in the fields of alpha-fetoprotein, CEA (carcinoembryonic antigen), isoenzymes and oncofetal antigens participated. It was an exciting event and it was followed in December 1974 by a Tokyo meeting sponsored by the New York Academy of Sciences (42) and by Drs. H. Hirai and E. Alpert, the organizers.

At the Tokyo meeting "Carcinofetal Proteins: Biology and Chemistry," close to 70 papers were presented by scientists from Japan, U.S.A., Finland, France, Singapore, Germany, Canada and Sweden. Dr. Hidematsu Hirai, Chairman of the Department of Biochemistry, Hokkaido University, was the recognized leader of the meeting. His large group of co-workers presented about half of the papers. In addition he had a radiant generous personality and was gracious in distributing alpha-fetoprotein specimens to all who requested this rare substance.

At a dinner hosted by the Tokyo meeting organizers, after all of us had enjoyed the sake and good food, I was asked to organize the next international meeting. I accepted because it was expected that the U.S.A. should be the venue of the next meeting and because the Tufts Cancer Research Center was the leading American institution committed to the oncodevelopmental concept. Also I was informed by telegram that we had received a high priority and approval for the renewal of the "Core" Center grant. The international meeting would bring favorable public recognition to Tufts Cancer Research Center and the University.

By the spring and summer of 1975, it became clear to me that it was not feasible to plan to have the meeting in Boston in view of the uncertainty of my future there. But where?

It so happened that I was appointed a Visiting Scientist for the month of February at the University of California at Los Angeles. Dr. Julien Van Lancker, head of its Pathology

Department, offered me the opportunity to collect placental specimens for Lil's and my studies on the developmental biology of the human placenta. We were able to travel to San Diego where I met with Dr. Stuart Sell of the University of California at San Diego (UCSD) whose laboratory was a major contributor to alpha-fetoprotein research. He was willing to cooperate if the next international meeting was to be in San Diego but was in no position to share responsibility for raising the necessary funds or for providing secretarial help.

We were impressed by La Jolla, the UCSD campus, the Salk Institute, and the Scripps Clinic and Research Foundation. When Lil said she could learn to like La Jolla, my reply was "then we will relocate the laboratory here." That settled the important question of where in California we would go.

In addition to Dr. Sell's laboratory, there were quite a number of investigators at the University, Salk, and Scripps who were engaged in one or more studies of carcinoembryonic proteins. The outstanding research activities of these institutes provided a stimulating environment into which I could transfer my laboratory from Tufts. We were going to move to La Jolla.

WHERE WAS THE SOURCE OF THE MONEY TO FUND THE SAN DIEGO MEETING?

There were several fundamental expenses to be met—the travel costs of the principal organizers of the Japanese meetings—travel allocations to overseas and domestic scientists, especially session chairmen—the cost of publishing the papers—the costs of organizing and administration of the meeting, etc. This was done by organizing a satellite conference in addition to the San Diego meeting.

The Kroc Foundation, established by Ray Kroc (Founder of McDonald's) in Santa Ynez, California, had sponsored a number of biomedical conferences and the National Cancer Institute often provided funding of conferences if matching funds could be committed by the applicant. Dr. Bob Kroc, the President of the Kroc Foundation, was willing to provide the matching funds. I had known Dr. Kroc for a number of years when he headed a research department at the Warner-Lambert Pharmaceutical Company in Morristown, New Jersey. If the applications were approved we would be able to reciprocate the treatment which the Japanese organizers had given us. The symposium we organized at Santa Ynez entitled "Regulation of Gene Expression in Development and Neoplasia," (43) won an NCI conference grant.

My plan was to have Drs. Hirai and Oda participate first in the San Diego meeting on "Oncodevelopmental Gene Expression" and then travel to Santa Ynez for the Kroc Conference. But who would publish these papers? *Cancer Research*, the official journal of the American Association for Cancer Research was willing to publish a supplement provided its page charges were met.

But how about the San Diego meeting? I wrote letters to and communicated with all the contacts I had in the pharmaceutical industry and in the health foundations. A key result was the decision of the Fannie E. Rippel Foundation to provide $10,000 for the publication of the papers of the San Diego meeting.

The San Diego Conference on "Oncodevelopmental Gene Expression" on May 23-28, 1976 was held in the Hotel del Coronado. Attendance was about 200. The National Cancer Institute co-sponsored the Kroc conference, and sufficient support from industry and academia was raised to cover all the expenses of both meetings.

How could the papers of the San Diego Conference be published in the shortest possible time? Academic Press, Inc. assured me that they could publish a hard cover volume three months after I provided them with "camera-ready" text. This

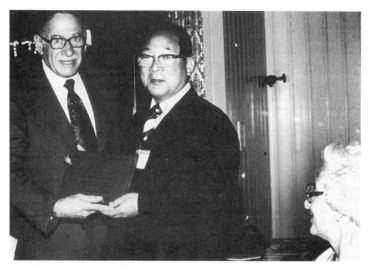

*San Diego Conference 1976 Award being presented to Professor Hidematsu Hirai
by Professor William H. Fishman at Hotel del Coronado*

would reduce publication time as there was no need to supply galley or page proof to the authors. The greatest uncertainty was the submission of the manuscripts which in the average case is a function of the procrastination or idiosyncrasy of a small number of our more or less egotistical but talented colleagues.

The speakers were notified that they would be required to submit their manuscripts to the chairman of their session. The manuscript would receive scientific review and a technical evaluation. We were lucky that Ms. Peggy Wilson edited each manuscript, obtained revisions from some of the speakers, and then transferred them to me. By the end of the meeting I had all the edited manuscripts in my possession and placed them in the hands of a printer who arranged "camera-ready" text. It took a total of five months from the end of the San Diego meeting for the hard-cover publication to appear (44). In the pre-laser computer printing days, this was a record.

Having decided to relocate to La Jolla, several important questions required answering. Would any of the existing research institutions be interested in providing or leasing laboratory space for my new venture? Would we have to set up a new Foundation to provide an approved mechanism for conducting research funded by the government? Should we buy a house now or wait till we got answers to the first questions? How should one effect an amicable separation from Tufts University School of Medicine? How about the careers of my staff?

We decided to set up a non-profit Foundation...but who was to do this? One day while looking through a brochure of the Scripps Clinic I noticed that their legal counsel was T. Knox Bell of Gray, Cary, Ames and Frye, a well-respected San Diego Law firm. Lil and I had a meeting with him scheduled after the Kroc conference. He undertook to prepare the Articles of Incorporation for a non-profit Foundation. What should it be called?

When I tried "Foundation for Oncodevelopmental Sciences" on my clinical friends, they shuddered and stated that the public would not understand its significance. "The La Jolla Cancer Research Foundation;" was the name chosen because the Foundation could serve as a coordinating central influence amongst the La Jolla institutions engaged in research and treatment of cancer. Two former Tufts colleagues, Dr. William Crosby, and Dr. Willard Vanderlaan were helpful in this very early phase of the creation of LJCRF.

Before and during the San Diego meeting, Lil was house-hunting in La Jolla. We were very fortunate in finding a house on the edge of a canyon with an ocean view and with sufficient land to garden. The unspoiled canyon is a delight to nature lovers and is inhabited by interesting wild life including opossums, foxes, raccoons, and skunks. Mocking birds and humming birds were numerous. We bought this house that week.

Lil and I returned to Boston with the satisfaction that both the San Diego and Santa Ynez meetings had gone well and that the papers of both would be published in 1976. In addition, the creation of the La Jolla Cancer Research Foundation was in progress and we had a home in La Jolla. We were on our way out of this "no-win" situation at Tufts.

GOODBYE TO TUFTS, HARRISON AVENUE, AND BOSTON

On my return to Boston, I learned that the Medical School belatedly had conferred tenure on me as Professor of Pathology...this after twenty-seven years of teaching and research and consistently passing all tests of peer review including that of the medical students. It was clear to me that the authorities had gotten wind of my search for a career opportunity elsewhere. They must have realized that were I to leave, there would be a considerable amount of grant funds which would be in jeopardy. I was not flattered by the late tenure award.

My first priority was to inform the Dean of my plans and to discuss the conditions of my departure. I told him that the La Jolla Cancer Research Foundation had recruited me as its President. If we could reach a mutually satisfactory agreement, he would have control of the space and operation of the Cancer Center three years earlier than scheduled. He would then have an immediate opportunity to appoint my successor and generate much more research funding. All I wished was to be given a terminal sabbatical year with salary. In my twenty-eight years at Tufts I had not taken off a single year of the four sabbaticals to which I was entitled. I also asked permission to transfer my NIH research grants and equipment purchased with those funds. He agreed but after leaving Tufts I ended up with a terminal sabbatical of six months, not a year! I was short-changed! I was permitted to transfer one NCI grant and relinquished the control of the Center grant.

BUT WHERE WAS THE RESEARCH TO BE DONE
IN LA JOLLA?

On July 9, 1976 the Articles of Incorporation of the La Jolla Cancer Research Foundation were issued by March Fong Eu, Secretary of State of California. Prior to this on July 4, I kissed Lil goodbye in Boston and announced that she would not see me again until I found a laboratory to which we could relocate our research activities.

I checked into a motel at La Jolla Cove and the next morning I walked along the shore. Imagine my astonishment to see live seals warming themselves on the rocks only 100 feet from shore. The surf pounding in was blue and clean in appearance. This contrasted with my former location near "skid row" and the "combat zone" of Boston which consisted of inner city sleaze and decay. To myself I said, this wonderful location is worth the gamble!

There were three institutions which were in a position to provide or lease laboratory space - the University, the Salk Institute and Scripps Clinic. Although there was some interest at the first two institutions, they had already organized their Cancer Centers. Scripps Clinic, however, was in the middle of a huge expansion on Torrey Pines Mesa and one of its buildings on South Coast Boulevard was becoming vacant. This was a 6000 sq. ft. apartment building which had been renovated into rather primitive lab space. The Clinic needed the cash income and we needed a laboratory. We negotiated a five-year lease at a very reasonable rental. So two weeks later I was on my way back to Boston with a letter of agreement to lease the apartment facility.

The question I asked Lil was—if we have a home in La Jolla and the laboratory also what are we doing in this house. The answer—sell it! The second couple to see our home in Brookline bought it.

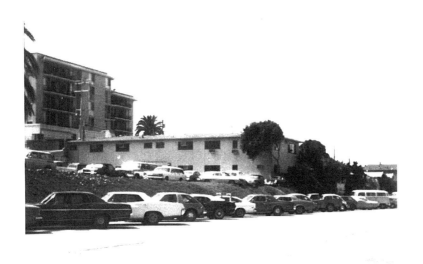

A view of the first home of the Foundation, 417 S. Coast Blvd., La Jolla

At this time, the staff of my laboratory consisted of two assistant professors, five post-doctoral students, four veteran technicians, one visiting scientist, and a number of technicians and students. Major equipment consisted of such instruments as a JEOL electron microscope, gamma counter, Beckman centrifuges, microscopes, autoanalyzers, etc. Staff members were all notified that I would help them relocate to La Jolla or elsewhere depending on their preferences. By September all of my staff were employed elsewhere. My administrative assistant, Sidney Green, decided to join the La Jolla Cancer Research Foundation. The visiting scientist, Dr. Shiro Iino, elected to complete his year in La Jolla.

The tradition had become established in academia that a scientist was permitted to transfer his grants and his equipment to the institution he was moving to. Tufts departed from this tradition. An inventory was made of all the equipment in my laboratory and the list circulated to various departments. Those could then select for their own use any item that appealed to them. As one could predict, the most modern and expensive equipment remained at Tufts—but that was the price I had to pay for my freedom. It was worth it.

MOVING TO LA JOLLA

We had an address to move to and a laboratory space for the Foundation. Two separate moves were coordinated. One was to load our personal belongings and furniture on a moving van and the other was to transfer the lab equipment and supplies to another van.

Our arrival in La Jolla preceded our furniture by two weeks. We lived in a motel for the first week and were able to move into our home by the second week. The furniture arrived on Labor Day weekend. We were able to occupy the 417 South Coast Boulevard premises by September 25. The lab materials arrived near October 1.

The transfer of our frozen specimens from Boston to San Diego was accomplished by packing them in dry ice, air-shipping them to San Diego, retrieving them from the air-freight terminal and storing them in a freeze-locker facility.

Our son, Daniel, arrived on Labor Day and we were happy to welcome his assistance. He served as office manager, public relations officer, inventory supply agent and in many other roles for three years. He then felt comfortable to resume his interrupted college education at San Diego State University. He graduated with distinction in Journalism and Advertising.

THE CANCER CENTER?

While all this was going on, my attention was focused on October 1, which was the NIH deadline for grant applications. It usually took nine months to a year from the time the application was submitted until, if approved with a high enough priority, it was funded. I prepared the application at home, using an outside secretarial service to complete it.

This was a "Planning Grant" for a Basic Science Cancer Center which requested $100,000 a year for two years to establish it. It was my great opportunity to define the scientific mission as the advancement of knowledge in the oncodevelopmental sciences and to outline the areas that merited attention. These included lab-clinical cooperation on the evaluation of tumor markers.

I also submitted a Program Project grant which was constructed along the lines of the Tufts "Core" grant, but which lacked individuals with ROI-NIH funding. It did include the efforts of Dr. Sell from UCSD, Dr. Gary David from Scripps, and Dr. Bill Crosby from the Scripps Clinic.

My hope was that by the time these applications were peer-reviewed, the components could be much more substantial and credible.

In the meanwhile we had to prepare for a National Cancer Institute management review of the Foundation. A team of accountants from the Washington NCI business office reviewed our administration to determine whether it could adequately monitor the grants and account for the funds being expended. They left satisfied and we were now accredited to administer NIH grants. My ROI grant at Tufts could now be transferred to La Jolla.

THE STAFF?

Two of my colleagues at the Tufts Cancer Research Center had committed themselves to join me in La Jolla. They each had their own ROI-grant and were important contributors to the oncodevelopmental idea. At the last minute, they reversed their decisions deciding that the risk of failure was too great for them.

In the meanwhile, I succeeded in recruiting Dr. Taiki Tamaoki of the University of Alberta at Edmonton for his sabbatical year. He saw this as an opportunity to compete for an NIH grant and to advance his career either in the USA or Canada.

Two of his postdoctoral students from Japan came with him. One was Dr. Shinzo Nishi, a member of Dr. Hirai's department of biochemistry at Hokkaido University and the other was Dr. K. Miura, from the pharmaceutical sciences faculty of Hokkaido University. Dr. Tamaoki's laboratory was experienced in the area of molecular biology as it related to the inverse expression of alpha-fetoprotein and albumin in neonatal development.

Dr. Shiro Iino, a gastroenterologist from the University of Tokyo had begun his studies with me in Boston. He rolled up his sleeves to help get the lab operating. For example, he constructed a table to support the Polaroid photographic equipment from a few boards with hammer and nails.

Lillian Fishman filled many important roles in those days. She was the purchasing agent, the equipment maintenance person, the lab manager in addition to conducting a research project with

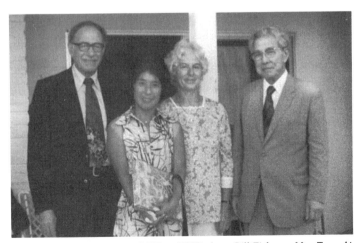

A visit with Professor Morizo Ishidate (1978) l to r Bill Fishman, Mrs. Tamaoki, Lil Fishman, Morizo Ishdate

Dr. Shiro Iino which yielded a publication (45). She was the Foundation's liaison with the community.

We were pleased to welcome Dr. Morizo Ishidate, who was our host in Japan 20 years earlier. He made a significant gift to the Foundation and expressed his admiration and support.

My role was that of Trustee, President, Scientific Director, Administrator and scientist. The challenge was to recruit additional competent staff so that some of my duties could be delegated.

PEER REVIEW

The Program Project grant was reviewed first. The site visit team included Dr. Erkki Ruoslahti, then at the City of Hope who later joined the Foundation. Representing the National Cancer Institute at that time was Dr. Brian Kimes from the Division of Cancer Biology. Before he left, he gave this advice to me "remember, we are happy to have you consult with us." The Program Project was structurally weak because it lacked a sufficient number of principal investigators with their own grants. It was regarded as too premature.

The site visit team for the cancer center planning grant consisted of Sidney Weinhouse, Robert Fahey, and Ernest Borek. They were enthusiastic about the oncodevelopmental approach and both Weinhouse and Borek had site-visited the Tufts Cancer Research Center in the past. The "pink sheets" indicated an excellent priority score two months later and we were elated at the news.

As the weeks went by, however, we learned that the Cancer Council had held up the funding. One of the members thought that there was a discrepancy in that our institution had submitted a Program Project which had a low score and a planning grant which excelled. The planning grant site visitors were asked to re-

review the application and submit a revised score. This review group resubmitted the same excellent fundable score as before. The Cancer Council was scheduled to make its decision a couple of weeks later. I flew to Washington and met with Dr. T. J. King, then the NCI Director and Dr. Brian Kimes of the Division of Cancer Biology. There was evidence of an apparent conflict of interest in the presence on the Council of an executive of a major La Jolla biomedical institute who was opposed to having another cancer center in La Jolla. I suggested to Dr. King that denying La Jolla Cancer Research Foundation the funding would constitute a major tragedy for the image of objectivity of the National Cancer Institute. He listened and excluded the member with an apparent conflict of interest from the next Council meeting.

The "planning grant" was funded and we had two years to produce a credible basic science cancer center. We were very happy!

The idea that an individual without adequate financial resources could create a scientifically respectable cancer research center in La Jolla in the presence of very powerful scientific research institutes struck many people as basically impossible. Word reached us that certain members of the staff at Scripps Clinic were betting that LJCRF would fold in six months at the latest. They lost their bets!

Cynicism was not a trait of Dr. John Spizizen, head of the biochemistry department at Scripps Clinic and Research Foundation. He had received his Ph.D. in Biochemistry from Toronto several years after I graduated. He was helpful in many ways and extended the hospitality of his laboratory to me and my staff. He served on our Board of Scientific Advisors for several years. In the Administration, I found Bob Erra, now Chief Financial Officer at Scripps, to be business-like and a pleasure to deal with. He leased the renovated apartment building to LJCRF at a reasonable rate.

RECRUITING STAFF

Two individuals joined my laboratory during the first year. One was Dr. Kimimaro Dempo, a pathologist from Sapporo Medical College. We studied the expression of several tumor markers in cancer of the lung. The other was Dr. José Luis Millán, a biochemist from Argentina who had won an International Rotary Club award to study in the U.S.A. He chose my lab and the field of oncodevelopmental isozymes. Several years after joining LJCRF, he met Dr. Torgny Stigbrand, a visiting scientist from the University of Umeå. José Luis directed the generation of monoclonal antibodies to isozymes of alkaline phosphatase which led to his being invited to do a Ph.D. thesis with Torgny in Umeå. José Luis became fluent in Swedish and indulged his love of music by singing in Swedish operas. By 1983, he received the "Doctor in Medical Science" degree. He has achieved recognition as an independent outstanding scientist. He is now a Senior Scientist at the Foundation. His laboratory has attracted scientists from Sweden, Japan, Switzerland, Belgium and Argentina. The torch of the research I carried to La Jolla has now been passed to him, successfully (46)!

It was also important to bring in talent in developmental biology. An especially attractive area was the study of mouse teratocarcinoma. From the participants at the Kroc conference, I learned of the competence of a young UCSF scientist named Elwood Linney. He needed support for the interval between submitting his own ROI grant application and its funding. LJCRF provided it. Another developmental biologist from Colorado, Cole Manes, was anxious to relocate and he brought his grant with him. His interest was in the early embryology of the rabbit. LJCRF also provided temporary appointments for two scientists who were abandoned after Microbiological Associates left San Diego. It was becoming very clear that we were greatly handicapped by the lack of good laboratory facilities...that our chances of attracting established investigators away from academia were very small. We prayed!

FACILITIES—ANSWER TO OUR PRAYERS

Dr. William Drell, President of Calbiochem, and I had known each other for some twenty-five years both professionally and personally. He agreed to become a Trustee of the La Jolla Cancer Research Foundation and donated $5000, a sum which was very significant to us at the time. Little did we anticipate that he would come up with a solution to our need for adequate facilities.

On the corner lot of North Torrey Pines Road and Science Park Road was a cancer research facility of Microbiological Associates. Sitting on close to five acres were two new buildings which had been designed for contract research to evaluate carcinogens and viruses. The management had expected to receive major funding from the National Cancer Institute, but shortly after the facility opened, NCI changed its policy and stopped this type of contract research. The owner of the property was the Whittaker Corporation in Los Angeles which found it could not afford the heavy losses of operating the Microbiological Associates facility. They decided to liquidate the facility, asking $3,000,000.

At about the same time, Calbiochem was sold to the Hoechst Corporation, a German firm with the status comparable to DuPont Corporation in the U.S.A. The California Foundation for Biochemical Research held Calbiochem shares which were called in, resulting in this organization receiving $2,000,000 in cash.

Bill Drell called me on the telephone and asked me if I was ready and willing to take on the Microbiological Associates facility if $2,000,000 was provided by his Foundation. The deal was that Whittaker Corporation would donate the land to the Foundation, California Foundation would contribute $2,000,000, and thus the Whittaker Corporation would achieve close to its selling price by virtue of the charitable deduction on the appreciated land plus the cash. LJCRF was required to administer the total lease and the rent would be 9.5% of $2,000,000 annually. This amount would then be a reasonable return on the investment by the California Foundation for Biochemical Research.

I did not hesitate for a second and accepted the challenge. The Trustees, however, had to approve this transaction. We met in a Conference Room in Bill Nelson's building on Prospect Street. One of our most highly regarded Trustees, Charles D. Doerr abstained from voting, saying that he feared I would suffer a heart attack from the extraordinary demands now about to be made on me. My answer was that I would suffer a heart attack if we didn't go ahead and acquire the facility. Since Dr. Drell and Mr. Doerr abstained, the vote was close with the Chairman, George C. Ellis, casting the deciding vote in favor of acquiring the facility.

THE MOVE TO TORREY PINES MESA

We had four months to end our lease on South Coast Boulevard and to move into the new facilities. This would mean a three-fold increase in the research laboratory space. How were we going to pay the rent? We inherited three tenants; Hanson Chemical, Becton-Dickinson and the ALS Foundation, all of whom moved out after a year. Hybritech moved into space leased back to the Whittaker Corporation and later into LJCRF space. However, our grant base was growing and between the rentals and the indirect costs reimbursement, we were able to meet the rent obligation. For several months, salaries and other obligations were not paid until the revenue caught up.

STRATEGIC PLANNING

We were in the second year of the planning grant and needed one more year before we could submit a credible "Core" grant application for a Cancer Center. We needed a first-class scientist who could be expected to fill the role of "Scientific Director". But who? Dr. Sell was not interested because of his satisfaction with his career at UCSD and the uncertain funding of LJCRF. I looked over the roster of members of the San Diego 1976 meeting and was convinced that Dr. Erkki Ruoslahti at the City of Hope was the best candidate. He had done excellent work on alpha-fetoprotein and was now engaged in the study of fibronectin, an adhesive protein important in embryonic cell migration. It so happened that in the Administration we had Dr. Robert Hasterlik who knew Dr. Ernst Beutler back at the University of Chicago. Dr. Beutler was taking an appointment at Scripps Clinic and Research Foundation, leaving the City of Hope. He brought us the news that Dr. Ruoslahti was unhappy at City of Hope and was looking to relocate. I telephoned Dr. Gene Roberts at City of Hope and he also told me that Ruoslahti was unhappy. He gave Ruoslahti a glowing recommendation. An invitation to speak at a seminar was dispatched quickly to Dr. Ruoslahti. He accepted and Drs. Ruoslahti and Engvall visited the Foundation. I asked Dr. Ruoslahti whether he would be interested in meeting the challenge of helping me create a Cancer Center. He was. It may have helped my case when I pointed out the parking lot as the site of a new building, if we found it necessary to build it.

But the City of Hope fought to keep Ruoslahti on their campus. They offered him a separate division of immunology, additional space and a big "hard money" budget. When I was informed of this counter-offer, I requested time to consult with our Trustees. From this came the final offer which included half the "hard money" budget of City of Hope, but a much more attractive long-term future. I even offered to build a tennis court on the Foundation grounds. To which Ruoslahti replied, "then you really are serious." He accepted the offer, minus the tennis court, with his move to take place by July 1, 1979.

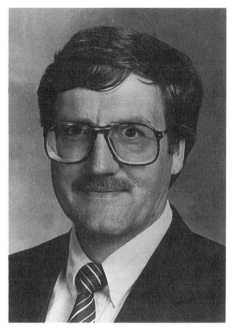

Dr. Erkki Ruoslahti, Scientific Director, 1979-1995, President 1989-

It so happened that both Ruoslahti and I attended a U.S.-Japan Conference in Honolulu in the spring. That was when we agreed on the planning of his laboratory space; his office was to be located next to mine. We also discussed the need for him to organize a program project, recruit one or two participants and to submit the application by October 1 that year.

THE GRAND OPENING

On January 18, 1979, the Foundation celebrated its move to Torrey Pines mesa and establishing itself as a neighbor to the Scripps Clinic, Salk Institute and UCSD. It was decided to tent the parking lot and to provide luncheon to all those who accepted the invitation. Amongst the speakers were Senator Joseph Biden, Dr. William Terry, Director of the NCI, and Dr. Jonas Salk, President of the Salk Institute. Faculty from our neighboring institutes were well-represented.

The following day we held the first Symposium of the Foundation in the North Building. This continues to be an annual prestigious event (see Appendix).

It was Bill Drell who commented at a Board of Trustees Meeting that we were witnessing a miracle on Torrey Pines Mesa... for Bill Fishman to have succeeded in less than two years in creating a credible cancer research center which was competitive with the best basic science cancer centers in the country.

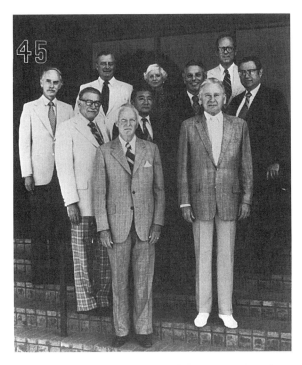

Board of Trustees, La Jolla Cancer Research Foundation, 1979. Back row (l. to r.) George Ellis, Chairman, Freddie (Broderick) Deming, Hal Taxel, Lou Cumming, Bill Drell. Front row (l. to r.) Jack Jaynes, Bill Fishman, Charles Doerr, T. Wakabayashi, Bert Aginsky

CHAPTER 13

GROWING PAINS

THE REVOLUTION

The Staff was drawn from highly diverse and individualistic backgrounds. The two scientists which were inherited, so to speak, from Microbiological Associates were Dr. Aaron Freeman, its Director and a Dr. David Kohne, a virologist. Dr. Freeman, transferred to the Foundation the residue of his grant funds and David Kohne, a one-year NIH contract. David Kohne had impressed Cole Manes and Elwood Linney with his technical expertise in DNA chemistry and the three constituted an entity that held its own seminars and did not share information with the rest of the staff. Dr. Francoise Farron-Furstenthal was an enzymologist from the Salk Institute previously known to us from Boston. Dr. Gary David came from Dr. Ralph Reisfeld's lab at Scripps and was working on the immunology of tumor markers.

The self-segregation of the Kohne, Manes and Linney trio led to their ambition to acquire the decision-making power of the Foundation. First they descended on Dr. Drell and expressed their dissatisfaction with Fishman's style, waving their club of considerable grant support they commanded. Then they tried to recruit a Philadelphia scientist who in my opinion was not suited for the overall scientific thrust of LJCRF. Next, they persuaded a trustee to be their voice in generating a direct link of the staff to the Trustees, by-passing the authority of the President. The Trustees then asked them to submit a revised set of by-laws for the Foundation. The Trustees rejected their proposal and registered their unanimous support for the President and the existing by-laws. The revolution was over.

Dr. Ruoslahti heard about this chaos and asked me if he still had a job at the Foundation. I assured him he did and that the Trustees supported me. Actually, a probable cause of the rebellion was the fear that their thrust for power would be ineffective once Ruoslahti came. I made up my mind that I was prepared for all of them to go and that Ruoslahti and I could recruit a much better staff and certainly a more loyal one.

What was lacking in the rebel staff was the understanding that authority has to be linked to responsibility. If the President makes a bad decision he is fired. If a committee of the staff decides an issue, no individual takes the negative consequences at all. As long as the President maintains communication and input from the staff, and reports back to them the Trustee decisions, he is fulfilling his obligation. The Trustees held the President responsible and accountable for the operation of the Institution. It follows that the staff was accountable to the President.

It so happened that the Site Visit for the third year of the planning grant was due. Drs. Ruoslahti and Engvall were to present their projects on extracellular matrix biochemistry as were each of the staff. One day before the site visit, Dr. Linney announced he was not going to participate. I quickly rearranged the agenda but felt outraged at the disloyalty of a scientist who had received so much support from the Foundation to launch his scientific career. It was very embarrassing. This was the event that motivated me to write in all the future employment contracts that the employee was required to cooperate for the welfare of the Institution. Lack of cooperation would be grounds for dismissal.

The revolution finally ended when I decided not to renew David Kohne's appointment once his contract term was over. Dr. Freeman moved to northern California, Dr. Linney to Duke University, and Dr. Farron-Furstenthal went into selling real estate. Dr. Manes joined the ALS Foundation and later became Professor and Chairman of the Biology department at the University of San Diego. This growing pain of the Foundation was now ended and a new era was in the offing.

THE CORE GRANT AND THE CANCER RESEARCH CENTER DESIGNATION

With Ruoslahti and Engvall on board, the scientific focus was directed to the extracellular matrix, its components and their role in cell interaction. Dr. Eileen Adamson brought the viewpoint of a biochemical embryologist and Dr. Robert Oshima the interest in teratocarcinoma and cytoplasmic cytokeratins. Dr. William Raschke from the Salk Institute was at the forefront of immunologic research on lymphocyte B-cells. Dr. Fishman's laboratory was active in research on oncodevelopmental enzymes and tumor markers. The Foundation and UCSD's department of pediatrics had signed a formal affiliation agreement to promote a study of the alpha-fetoprotein tumor marker in hepatoblastoma. Altogether, we were able to define for the Center a credible scientific mission in oncodevelopmental biology which reached out to our neighboring institutes.

At the same time Dr. Ruoslahti had put together an outstanding program project on the extracellular matrix whose other participants were Eva Engvall, Charles Birdwell, Ed Hayman, and Eileen Adamson.

Both the Core Grant and the Program Project were evaluated by separate peer-review teams and both were awarded high funding priorities. The terms of these awards was three years. The Foundation was now an NCI-designated Basic Science Cancer Research Center, a credential which only two other California Institutions shared—The Salk Institute and the California Institute of Technology.

The great satisfaction to us was that we had succeeded in

creating an institution whose primary commitment was to advance knowledge in the related sciences of developmental biology and cancer—the oncodevelopmental concept. The top priority of the operation was to produce an environment in which scientists could thrive and in which administration was there to serve the scientists. Lil and I firmly believed that the life of LJCRF depended on its sending roots into the community of La Jolla and San Diego. It could not prosper long as "a foreign body" in this region no matter how great the scientific credentials.

THE "COMMUNITY" AND LJCRF

Several communities could be recognized. First, there were our own friends and relatives in the US and Canada; next, there was the population of first-class scientists here and elsewhere especially in NCI-designated cancer centers; then there were the Trustees of the La Jolla Cancer Research Foundation; the Presidents Council and finally, the public at large.

Prior to the visit of the NCI Management Review Site Visit, only three months after we moved into 417 S. Coast Blvd., it was necessary to show evidence of community support. Letters were written to all our friends and relatives and they were invited to become the first friends of LJCRF. There was a good response. A surprise was a donation of $1000 from Mr. H. Leland, a distant relative on my mother's side unknown to me and a pledge for four more such annual gifts. It turns out that the Lelands had lost a son to cancer. Dr. and Mrs. Drell generously donated $5000, an amount that overwhelmed us.

It was decided that a newsletter should be written and edited by Lil and distributed every month to those on the Foundation list of attendees to all its events. This list was to grow reaching four thousand by 1989. Lil's effort was to translate the research program into a narrative that could be understood and appreciated by the average reader of the newsletter. She was successful.

The main expenses of the newsletter were printing costs, paper and postage. Assembly of the newsletter, labeling, folding, and sorting was carried out by a band of loyal volunteer members of the Friends group. Lil transported the newsletters to the Post Office herself, all packaged by zip code. In the last few years of her editorship, a mailing company did the mailing. The participants in this enterprise included Mr. and Mrs. Herman Silberman, Beverly Mungle, Mary Wall, Bonnie Kane, and many others.

Donors who had never seen the Foundation were attracted to it by the human interest events reported in the monthly Newsletter. Thus, one day Mr. Thornton walked in with $20,000 of South African Krugerrands gold coins. His wife willed them to the Foundation because she believed from her reading the Foundation Newsletter over the years that the Foundation merited the bequest. Similarly, Ms. Anita Martin has for the same reason willed the Foundation all of her estate.

With the growth in the number of volunteers and in recognition of their loyalty and enthusiasm, Freddy Deming and Lil created the "Friends of LJCRF" organization. A set of by-laws was written which were approved by the Board of Trustees and membership defined. Before long there were over one hundred members. Their goal was to raise money for specialized equipment.

In 1980 we had a pressing need for a Hitachi combined scanning and transmission microscope which was priced at $250,000. Application was made to NIH for half of this amount since equipment grants required a matching sum from the institution. The rest had to be raised by the Foundation. To the Trustees this was an unprecedented obligation. With great reluctance they approved fund-raising in the amount of $125,000 as a goal, not a commitment. A committee was appointed, headed by Milton Cheverton to try to raise this intimidating amount.

The Friends did not hesitate one minute. They scheduled fund-raising art auctions, galas, rummage sales in short order and raised $25,000. At this juncture, I ordered the electron microscope. California Foundation pledged substantial support as did individual business firms. We were lucky. Before the instrument was delivered the NIH funded the matching grant and the Foundation succeeded in raising the rest of the funds. Also we were fortunate to recruit George Klier, a talented electron microscopist to manage this important facility. His work was highly regarded in the scientific community.

How did the Foundation attract volunteers? The following story is an example:

During the early years of the Foundation, San Diego's radio station, KFMB, featured a commentator named Harold Kean. He would interview people in the news. The Friends were organizing an Art Auction to help pay for the electron microscope and word reached KFMB and I was invited to be interviewed to gain publicity for our event. It so happened that a candidate for Congress, Duncan Hunter, was also interviewed the same evening. He was elected and still holds office in Washington. (His sister, Bonnie Kane, later became a strong supporter of the Friends of LJCRF.)

The next morning, two ladies showed up at the Foundation who stated they had heard me being interviewed by Harold Kean and they wanted to help. They were Beverly Mungle and Mary Wall.

Beverly Mungle was the cheerful "can-do" type who became a dedicated member of the Friends group. She was most generous and kind to her co-workers and operated a type of shuttle service, calling for elderly members who lacked cars and bringing them to and back from Friends' meetings and events.

Mary Wall originally from Australia, exuded competence and confidence. She likewise devoted herself to the fund-raising activities of the Foundation. She possessed a lively intellect and a great sense of humor. With her passing in 1990, she left the Foundation over $50,000 from her estate. This gift has been recognized by the naming of a Conference Room in the new building in her memory.

That San Diego has citizens such as Beverly Mungle and Mary Wall, bodes well for its deserving not-for-profit organizations.

Subsequent fund-raising drives were focussed on the need for sophisticated equipment such as the amino acid synthesizer and the amino acid sequencer, the DNA oligonucleotide sequencer and synthesizer, The Finnegen Mass Spectrometer, start-up equipment for new investigators, etc. were all purchased from funds raised in large part by the Friends.

Most memorable was the leadership of Patricia Carlson in conceiving and conducting two galas based on the "Sentimental Journey" theme. The same success was achieved with three successive "Magical Experiences" which drew a lot of favorable attention to the Foundation, the last being chaired by Junko and Larry Cushman.

Headquarters for all of the above activities was centered in Lil's office. A more detailed description of the Friends' activities is given in on pages 167-70.

CHAPTER 14

MY VIEWS OF CANCER RESEARCH

In 1946, it was in the Department of Surgery at the University of Chicago that I first became acquainted with cancer—human cancer specimens. The usual experience of the biochemist doing cancer research was to work on transplanted hepatoma cells in mice of the same genetic background. These transplanted hepatomas grew very rapidly and provided grams of tumor tissue per mouse. This tissue was ground up in a homogenizer and samples could then be subjected to the analysis of one or more constituents or functions. Although the biochemist thus could have the convenience of harvesting a uniform population of tumor cells, the interpretation of the results could not be precise nor specifically relevant to cancer. After many transplant generations, the tumor cells lost many of the identifying characteristics of the original tumor. Consequently it was never certain whether the phenomena observed could be attributed simply to cell proliferation or to a unique tumor cell proliferation.

Throughout the years I found that the field was dominated by the "high priests" of biochemistry whose experimental technology was very demanding. It was accepted that the most meaningful results could be secured only through mastering the most intricate techniques.

The best example of this was the monopoly of cancer research from 1930 to 1960 by the Nobel Prize winner, Otto Warburg. The centerpiece of all these researches was the Warburg manometric apparatus which consisted of two banks of seven manometers with vessels containing tissue materials and buffers; the latter being immersed in a constant temperature bath. All vessels and manometers had to be carefully calibrated and each vessel could be attached to only one manometer; none were interchangeable. The noise of the moving banks of manometers, the necessity to record manually the rate of change in the mercury level in each manometer, the agility required of the experimenters all combined to impress the observer that the most significant research was in progress. It is understandable that scientists who had mastered the Warburg apparatus; who had invested so much in acquiring the equipment and who accepted the opinions of the great Warburg without a question would not easily relinquish this technology. It always produced results but not necessarily significant interpretations.

Warburg's studies (47) led him to theorize that an injury to a cell's ability to respire caused it to compensate by increasing fermentation in order to generate the cell's energy requirement. This process caused the cell to become malignant. I remember arguing with my colleagues that the energy dynamics of the cell were far distant from the actual cause of cancer. I drew the analogy of a locomotive pulling a string of box cars, stating that it made little difference what fuel provided the energy for the locomotive, the train would still move forward. The cause of cancer must be much more subtle, I believed.

The above example illustrates how a number of scientists have characterized my thinking. Dr. Camillo Artom at the Bowman-Gray School of Medicine told me—"Bill, you think like a peasant." This opinion was a compliment as I interpreted it to mean that I was able to go to the heart of the problem directly. In my own way, I was postponing acceptance of views of the origin of cancer advanced by famous spokesmen from prestigious institutions until they registered with me as fundamental plausible ideas.

As it turned out, Dr. Sidney Weinhouse, in 1972, through the detailed study (41) of the known metabolic pathways with the use of isotopically labeled intermediates came to the conclusion that no defect could be demonstrated in the cancer cell's respiratory equipment. The explanation of the increased respiration in some tumors was due to the role of fetal isozymes of respiration which became dominant in cancer cells. According to Dr. Henry Pitot (48), this could be a phenomenon consequent to the progression of a cell to malignancy but certainly not its cause.

A similar attempt at a unitary hypothesis of cancer was the "Convergence Theory" of Dr. Jesse Greenstein (49), once Director of the Biochemistry Division of the National Cancer Institute. This held sway from 1943 to 1953. It contended that the direction of all cancer cells was to achieve a common enzyme pattern. This was the consequence of measuring a number of enzyme activities in transplanted multi-generation hepatomas. It was uncritically accepted since it seemed to accord so well with Warburg's views and research; and Warburg was the high priest.

A variety of "deletion" hypotheses held sway for decades afterwards. The first was the interpretation of the Miller and Miller experiments (50) in 1947. They observed that the carcinogen (azo dye) bound specifically to certain proteins in the cytoplasm of normal liver cells. There was a consequent absence of these proteins in the resulting hepatoma cells. The deletion of these proteins led the cells to compensate by proliferating out of control was their explanation. This last inference was also accepted uncritically even though cell proliferation is only one feature of malignant cells.

Over the years the view was prevalent that if the study was "good biochemistry", then it was automatically "good cancer research". This view floundered with the emergence of the concepts that cancer was a disease of development, involved the re-expression of fetal genes and the balance between oncogenes and tumor suppressor genes.

In 1967, Dr. G. Barry Pierce (51) postulated that cancer was a phenomenon rooted in developmental biology. This idea (44) grew out of his work on mouse teratocarcinomas which could be generated from early embryonic cells and Mintz and Illmensee (52) demonstrated the ability of teratocarcinoma cells to function as normal embryonic cells when the former was introduced into the blastocyst.

Three discoveries brought the oncodevelopmental concept to the attention of cancer researchers. In 1963, Dr. G. I. Abelev (37) and Y. Tatarinov (38) independently demonstrated the re-expression in mouse and human cancer cells of the embryonic liver alpha-fetoprotein (AFP). In 1965, Drs. Gold and Freeman (39) reported the presence of carcinoembryonic antigen (CEA) in colon cancer and the Fishman laboratory discovered a placental alkaline phosphatase (PLAP) in the cancer cells and blood serum of a patient with terminal lung cancer. Today there is no aspect of oncogenes or tumor suppressor genes which is not related to processes of developmental biology. This also applies to "apoptosis", programmed cell death, which is a necessary phenomenon in embryologic development.

From my perspective, the biochemical fads of the past did not survive the test of time and the different causes of cancer (chemical carcinogens and x-ray damage, etc.) each was given a separate explanation.

By 1975, because of the great advances in cloning and sequencing genes, it had been agreed that the primary target of cancer producing agents was DNA, the hereditary substance in the nucleus of cells which is the residence of all the genes we inherited from our parents. Such genes could undergo mutation and in circumstances which favor the sequential "turning-on" of oncogenes interspersed with the "turning-off" of tumor suppressing genes, the process could proceed from initiation to progression to neoplasia and to metastasis.

THE RIDDLE OF CANCER IS BEING SOLVED!

Perhaps because of my first experiences with human cancer at the University of Chicago(15), I was influenced to relate my discoveries in basic research to human cancer. Thus, having established in mice that the enzyme ß-glucuronidase was correlated with the action of steroid hormones, we were motivated to interpret the relatively high values in human cancer tissues as a reflection of this action. This, in turn, led us to investigate the ß-glucuronidase concentration in the vaginal and cervical fluids of women with cancer of the cervix. The major result of clinical value actually turned out to be the ß-glucuronidase enrichment of spinal fluid by brain tumors, a tumor marker.

Next at Tufts in 1953, we developed a tumor marker test for prostate cancer based on a new technique of measuring the acid phosphatase isozyme of prostatic origin (24). It became the standard test for two decades and was superseded by a radioimmunoassay for prostatic acid phosphatase.

Finally, the basic research on the isoenzymes of alkaline phosphatase led to the separate measurement of the bone, liver, intestinal, and placental isoenzymes in serum. This achievement being further refined by others since has been of major clinical value in defining the tissue source of the isozymes in sera of patients with many disorders including cancer (53).

The production of the placental isozyme by cancer tissue has led to sophisticated successful radioimmunolocalization and radioimmunotherapy of cancers of the ovary by Epenetos in London (36).

It has been the clinical value of some of our findings which has given me the satisfaction to know that I have kept the bargain which the citizens of this country made with its scientists when they supplied the funds for our cancer research.

CHAPTER 15

THE INTERNATIONAL SOCIETY FOR ONCODEVELOPMENTAL BIOLOGY AND MEDICINE (ISOBM)

In Sapporo located in Hokkaido, the northern island of Japan, Dr. Hidematsu Hirai had organized a team of investigators who focused their research on all aspects of alpha-fetoprotein (AFP). They prepared AFP in pure form and supplied samples to investigators from many countries. These served as standards for analytical immunoassay methods.

In the fall of 1973, Drs. H. Hirai and T. Wada hosted a conference in Sapporo to which a number of these scientists were invited plus others active in the studies of CEA and the Regan Isozyme.

Dr. Hirai was a heavy-set, high-energy individual with a great deal of charm. Moreover, he really was the leader in Sapporo and in all of Japan in this tumor marker area. The greatest attention was paid to these proteins as tumor markers and the group compared results obtained in different countries with similar populations of cancer patients. We were about twenty attendees and our hosts extended wonderful hospitality including banquets and a bus tour to the countryside. We named ourselves "The International Research Group for Carcinoembryonic Proteins."

We were all pleased to learn that Dr. Hirai and Dr. Elliot Alpert were planning a major 1974 meeting in Tokyo under the auspices of the New York Academy of Sciences. This would give us an opportunity to prepare our most interesting work for presentation. Thus it was in December, 1974, that some two hundred scientists gathered to present forty-seven papers which were subsequently published the following year in the *Annals of the New York*

Academy of Sciences (42). It seemed clear that the Japanese should not be expected to host the future meetings and so, as I have reported earlier, we undertook the job of hosting the next meeting in the United States.

The San Diego meeting was historic both for its significance to the raison d'être of the La Jolla Cancer Research Foundation and for the consensus that here was the beginnings of a new scientific society. The rapid publication of *"Onco-Developmental Gene Expression"* (42) and the monograph (41) in *Cancer Research* of "Regulation of Gene Expression in Development and Cancer" widely disseminated the new information and broadened the perspective from "tumor markers" *per se* to the contribution they could make defining more clearly the precise nature of cancer.

DR. HIDEMATSU HIRAI

Dr. Hirai, who was the President of the Society until he died in 1991, was its moving force and made all the decisions albeit after consultation with the parties concerned. At the annual meetings, he also generated a good feeling of camaraderie amongst the membership, singing folk songs in Japanese, German, and English and encouraging others to sing their country's folk songs.

Dr. Hirai's friendship and help were invaluable in the formative years both of the Foundation and the Society. He permitted his department member, Dr. Shinzo Nishi to accompany Dr. Tamaoki to La Jolla. He officially named the La Jolla Cancer Research Foundation as the United States Regional Center of the Society. We worked closely in identifying the future organizers of the Society meetings and in providing them some financial support and advice. He depended on me to develop the by-laws of the Society. He was able to attract significant financial support for the Society from the Japanese government and pharmaceutical industry. He served on our Board of Scientific Advisors and participated in a Core Grant site visit.

He did appreciate that through my effort he became more visible in the West as a leader of oncodevelopmental biology. This was a consequence of the San Diego and Kroc meetings.

We did have one serious difference of opinion. In 1982, Elsevier Press decided it would not continue publication of the Society's Journal and offered to transfer its files and rights to the next publisher. At Hirai's request I made a thorough survey of potential publishers and ended up with several prospects. The most interested of these was Liss Publishing Company, New York, whose specialty was the publication of journals with modest circulation numbers. They provided me with a formal proposal which had advantageous terms for the Society. That Fall there was another ISOBM meeting in Sapporo and the Editorial Board reviewed the proposals. It voted for Liss as the publisher and instructed me to complete the arrangements. I was looking forward to having more control of editorial policy and its standards in order that the journal should reflect the scientific quality of the Society. Imagine my chagrin when Hirai conveyed a message to Liss that his proposal was disapproved. Instead a Japanese publisher was engaged, the name of the journal was changed to *Tumour Biology* without my input. There was now a choice I was compelled to make. Either I would contest Hirai's arbitrary decision at a special Board meeting or I would not. I decided not to and to resign my position as Editor. This way I could maintain my friendship with Hirai since we would not have to engage further in a power struggle over control of the philosophy of the journal, which indeed it was.

My earlier efforts to upgrade the journal ran into a cultural difference with Dr. Hirai. My view was that merit only should be the yardstick for accepting manuscripts for the journal. Hirai's view was that every member of the Society should have the right to have his or her manuscript accepted. In Japan, at that time, one view was that the Editor was honor-bound to accept a manuscript submitted by a colleague, no matter how poor its quality. Dr. A. Munro Neville who succeeded me as co-editor accepted this philosophy and turned over to Dr. Aaron Malkin, the Managing Editor, most of the day-to-day responsibilities of the Journal.

RECOLLECTION OF SOME ISOBM MEETINGS

The Sapporo Symposium on Carcinoembryonic Proteins was held in Japan, October 23 and 24, 1973. It was organized by Dr. Hidematsu Hirai, Professor of Biochemistry, Hokkaido University and by Dr. Takeo Wada, Professor of Medicine, Sapporo Medical College. The Symposium was a consequence of the widespread realization that the re-expression of alpha-fetoprotein, an embryonic yolk sac protein, in hepatoma patients provided a significant tumor marker. Dr. Hirai's laboratory became a center for the preparation and distribution of this tumor marker protein. This resulted in new information which Dr. Hirai collected annually and distributed in newsletter form. In Japan, hepatoma was a major cause of deaths from cancer and this explains why sixty of sixty-six attendees were Japanese biomedical researchers. The non-Japanese present were Drs. Alpert, Fishman, Gitlin, Kohn, Masseyeff, and Simons.

It is of historical interest to examine the session topics— Ontogeny of Fetal Plasma Proteins, Chemistry of Alpha-Fetoproteins, Detection Method of AFP, Experimental Hepatoma, Pathology of Liver Diseases and AFP, HB(Au)-Antigen and Hepatoma, Carcinoembryonic Enzymes, and Clinical Aspects of Carcinoembryonic Proteins.

And to compare them with the sessions in Sapporo of the 20th Anniversary meeting in 1992 of the International Society for Oncodevelopmental Biology and Medicine. These were

Cancer Associated Mucin Antigens, Molecular Aspects of the CEA family, Cell Adhesion Molecules in Cancer, Clinical Aspects of Tumor Markers, Cell Growth and Differentiation, Tumor Related Genes and Products and Immunoscintigraphy and Immunotherapy. Some 430 names were listed in the Author Index; many coming from the USA, Europe, Russia, Middle East and, of course, Japan. The meeting took four days.

In November 1974, the next important meeting took place in Tokyo preceded by a closed AFP Symposium in Nice organized by Dr. R. Masseyeff. The Tokyo meeting was held under the auspices of the New York Academy of Science and the International Research Group for Carcinoembryonic Proteins. The organizers were Drs. Hidematsu Hirai and Elliot Alpert. Attendance from the U.S. and Europe was significant and the Conference papers were published in the *Annals of the New York Academy of Sciences* "Carcinofetal Proteins: Biology and Chemistry". It was there that I accepted the responsibility of hosting the next international meeting, the story of which has been detailed earlier.

The goal of the San Diego meeting in 1976 was to attract the attention of the biomedical scientific community in the USA to this new field of cancer research. The satellite Kroc Conference was to achieve a sharper focus of the key issues.

It became clear to me that it had become necessary to coin a term for this field which could be adequate into the foreseeable future. Thus, "oncofetal antigens" was really an immunologic definition; "Carcinoembryonic Proteins" could be mistaken for "Carcinoembryonic Antigens (CEA)". These tumor markers all had their counterparts in fetal development. Eventually, "oncodevelopmental biology" was suggested and it first became nationally visible with the publication of the San Diego meeting "Oncodevelopmental Gene Expression". The result for a time was a convergence of the interests of the La Jolla Cancer Research

Foundation and the yet to be established scientific society. The more visible and significant the field of oncodevelopmental biology became, the more relevant became the "raison d'être" of the Foundation.

The meeting was a memorable one. The setting at the Hotel del Coronado was unique. This was a hotel built in the 1880s which was the choice of the wealthy and the famous over the decades, providing an exclusive beach on an island which was reached by a beautiful bridge spanning San Diego harbor. Half way through the meeting there was an out-of-doors picnic luncheon at the San Diego Zoo with a report on its research program by Dr. Kurt Benirshke. It was funded by Bill Drell's Calbiochem company. At the banquet, Awards of Merit were presented to Dr. Hidematsu Hirai and to Dr. Phil Gold for their pioneer studies on AFP and CEA, respectively. Dr. G. I. Abelev received an award of Merit *in absentia*.

At the business meeting, LJCRF was designated as the North American headquarters of the International Research Group.

In 1977, the Group held a meeting in Copenhagen organized by Dr. Bengt Norgaard-Pederson. It honored Professor Teilum for his work on yolk sac testicular tumors which produced AFP. In Copenhagen the Council agreed to plan the organization of a formal scientific society which would publish its own journal.

The plan was presented the following year in Marburg, Germany at the annual meeting organized by Dr. Frank G. Lehmann. I served as Chairman of both the by-laws and journal committees. The well attended meeting (over four hundred) approved the proposals and so was born the International Society for Oncodevelopmental Biology and Medicine. Dr. Lehmann who had solicited proposals from several publishers presented the winning one, Elsevier Press. He was appointed the Managing Editor and lived long enough to see the first year of publication. He died from a disseminated renal carcinoma. I visited him on my way to the Moscow meeting in 1980 and took over the responsibilities of the managing editor.

The meeting in Sussex, U.K., in 1979 was chaired by A. Munro Neville, Director of the Cancer Center at the Royal Marsden Hospital. His colleague Iochim (Jim) Kohn was doing his best to integrate his boss into the leadership of the Society. Thus, Munro succeeded Frank Lehmann as the Managing Editor of the Journal and in 1992, followed Dr. Hirai as the Editor. The meeting itself was held on the grounds of Sussex University and was the scene of the first reports by Goldenberg and by Mach of targeting colon cancer with radioactive monoclonal antibodies to CEA.

In all of the Society's meetings before 1987, Dr. Gari Abelev was not an attendee by virtue of the Soviet Union's policy of repressing individual's freedom to travel. Abelev had refused to censure a colleague who had taken steps to emigrate to Israel. Consequently, he was denied travel outside of Russia. However, he and his colleagues were determined to hold a meeting in Russia. This is how it was done in 1981.

The organizer of the meeting was Dr. Trapeznikov, Director of the All-Union Cancer Center in Moscow. Dr. Abelev and Tatarinov were listed inconspicuously in the scientific committee. It was decided not to hold the meeting in Moscow because of its saturation with KGB personnel. In Tallinn, Esthonia, Dr. V. I. Ryatsep, a clinical oncologist, headed the meeting which was as far from Moscow as possible. The big problem for attracting participants from the U.S. and Europe was that U.S.S.R. had invaded Afghanistan and many scientists had canceled their attendance to meetings in the U.S.S.R. as a protest against the invasion. My concern was for the position of our hosts if no Americans came to the Tallinn meeting. They would suffer hostility and reprisals from the USSR academic power structure. I decided to go. One other American, Elliot Alpert, also attended.

It was the first time I met Dr. Abelev and Dr. Tatarinov.

Abelev was a short, stout, very intense individual who clearly knew every detail of the several research papers his younger colleagues delivered. I presented him with the San Diego meeting Award for Merit in my hotel room. He was very appreciative. He clearly was a kind gentle human being who bore his suffering from political adversity quietly.

Dr. Tatarinov, who had first demonstrated AFP in human hepatoma was an extrovert, on the other hand. He delighted in singing Russian folk songs and in dancing with enthusiasm to both folk music and modern jazz.

The route to Tallinn was via Moscow. Dr. Abelev arranged for one of his younger colleagues, Dr. Eugene Mechetner, to meet me at the airport and to be my guide (and my protector) in Moscow. When he drove apparently through a red light in the Lenin Hills, site of Moscow University, he was stopped by a uniformed policeman. I thought we were now in real trouble. I could be accused of being an American CIA agent. Eugene opened his luggage door, took out a half-liter bottle of laboratory alcohol, gave it to the officer and we went on our way—not even a traffic ticket.

That evening was the night before Yom Kippur, the Day of Atonement, the holiest day of the year to us Jews. Eugene guided me to the Grand Synagogue of Moscow. A crowd was gathered at the steps and I assumed all the seats were taken…when I noticed that a man was motioning me to follow him. I did and assumed Eugene was behind me. To my surprise, I was ushered to an area close to the Ark where there were several chairs. The Synagogue was ablaze with light and completely filled. A choir of six Cantors thrilled the congregation with their opera-like renditions of the prayers. Afterwards when I offered New Years greetings and extended my hand, there was no one who took it. This all became understandable when I learned that my seat in the Synagogue was in an area reserved for foreigners and that no one dared to have physical contact with them because of the scrutiny of the KGB. The person who motioned for me to follow him on my arrival was identified as a KGB agent. On my way out, I found Eugene standing in the back. He was not permitted to accompany me to the foreigners area.

Subsequent meetings of ISOBM continued annually without interruption as follows: 1981 Banff, Canada; 1982 Sapporo, Japan; 1983 Stockholm, Sweden; 1984 Houston, U.S.A.; 1985 Paris, France; 1986 Helsinki, Finland; 1987 Quebec, Canada; 1988 Barcelona, Spain; 1989 Freiburg, Germany; 1990 Moscow, U.S.S.R.; 1991 Sienna, Italy; 1992 Sapporo, Japan and in 1993 Jerusalem, Israel.

In the course of these meetings, the name of the journal was changed to *Tumour Biology* and the Publisher now is S. Karger. At each meeting advances in cancer research were reviewed and many international collaborative studies were initiated.

CHAPTER 16

EVOLUTION OF THE ADMINISTRATIVE STRUCTURE AND SCIENTIFIC PROGRAMS

Several principles guided us. One was to impose the very minimum of bureaucracy on the staff, to have the administration serve the scientists' needs and to provide accountability to the Board of Trustees. Finally, the buck stops with the President!

The history of the assembly of the LJCRF administration has its beginnings at Tufts. Sidney Green first worked as a technician with me in the early 1950s on a variety of problems. He was assigned responsibilities later which centered on management of the laboratory and working with relevant officials of the Medical School administration. As a co-author and laboratory liaison he was valuable and carried with him the laboratory memory of analytical procedures which contributed to the continuity of effort. His background as a clinical chemist was important in organizing and conducting lab/clinical joint projects. He mastered the "Autotechnicon" apparatus which was the pioneer in automated clinical analyses and it became central to the performance of our clinical projects. He accompanied the scientific staff to all the Federation Meetings and participated in discussions. However, his effort to acquire an advanced degree in biochemistry met with failure and consequently, he learned on-the-job to be a laboratory manager.

When in 1976, I explained to him my plan to relocate to the La Jolla Cancer Research Foundation, he was eager to join, pledging to do his share of income generation through a "tumor marker" laboratory tests service - around $100,000 a year. He demanded the title of Vice-President and a salary greater than the President's. He got the title but not the salary. No "tumor marker" laboratory was ever created.

This was a classical case of the "Peter Principle"—where an individual is promoted to a position far beyond his competence although he was sent to San Diego State University where he completed a course in management. Unfortunately there was no instruction in judgement. Thus, as our funds in the first year were diminishing rapidly, he paid all the invoices as soon as we received them. It didn't occur to him that the discount on early payment of our bills wasn't any advantage if our cash flow ceased. On that occasion, he took a draft of the monthly statement to Cole Manes and alarmed him. This set in motion demands from Manes, Linney, and others for assurances that the Foundation could meet its financial obligations and that their research and their careers were not in jeopardy. Sid's action was taken without my knowledge.

I decided to recruit a management consultant who would evaluate our operation and who would provide us recommendations. He, Mr. Samuel Katz, interviewed each member of the staff. He concluded that we had to improve the communications between the parties and suggested I preside over a management committee made up of Cole Manes, Sid Green, and Lil and to meet weekly. This mechanism proved to be very useful and it was utilized from that time till 1989 when I relinquished the presidency.

The operations committee was expected to bring up for consideration any event or plan which could affect the health of the Foundation. There was no penalty for complaints and so the President's awareness of new or recurrent problems was never more than one week late. Moreover, the managers of the various components of the administration knew that they had equal access to the President if they thought it necessary.

By the time of the 1983 renewal of the Core Grant, the

Foundation had a qualified Administrator, Ken Lasbury, to whom Sid Green reported as a grants manager, relinquishing the title of Vice-President. This grants management area was one in which Green was well-qualified. The NCI site visitors were favorably impressed with our administration and the progress made in developing the scientific program.

Over the years a solid and responsible infrastructure was built. The accounting office was headed by competent Sally Sullivan who maintained good communication with each staff scientist and provided them a monthly report. She developed a good esprit de corps amongst her staff, one of whom, Sherri Marinovich, eventually ended up as the director of the Human Resources department of LJCRF. Jennifer East, a bundle of energy and intelligence organized the purchasing office in such a way, that the orders submitted by staff were processed in the shortest possible time. Carl Crader started off as Chief of Maintenance but very soon demonstrated excellent ability to undertake any and all renovations which were needed to accommodate the scientists. He literally saved the institution many thousands of dollars. Rob Shaw served as the safety officer and monitored all the laboratories for radioactive and other spills.

A number of committees of the Board of Trustees served both to monitor certain key areas of activity and to report to the Chairman of the Board and the President. The Finance Committee reviewed the monthly financial statements, the annual budget and the management of funds. The Chairman of this committee was always the treasurer of LJCRF. The Development Committee oversaw the fund raising, social events, and capital fund drives. The Building Committee monitored the construction of a new building and the library. The Science Committee participated in the annual meeting of the Board of Scientific Advisors which reviewed the scientific program and the records of staff to be considered for promotion.

These Trustee committees completed the communication loop between staff, Administration, and Trustees.

Community participation was identified with the Trustees and their role as ambassadors of the Foundation. The various fund-raising events which Lil and Freddie Deming and others put on were attended by Trustees and their friends resulting in the "family" feeling which became a characteristic of the institution. The site visit reports were congratulatory on the evidence of community support which LJCRF had gathered.

Lil and I had always placed a high priority on developing good relations with the community. We placed a lot of weight on the monthly Newsletter which Lil edited. It was distributed to all donors and relevant academic and industrial institutions. In this way, the human interest profiles on our new staff and new Trustees appeared in each issue along with one science report written in a clear intelligible style.

No one knows what triggers an impulse to donate money to the Foundation. It is not enough that the Institute has a good scientific reputation, though it helps… as does a prestigious Board of Trustees. In some cases, the loss of a loved one to cancer leads one to seek a way to fight back.

This is the story of Sam (Rush) Spaulding of Los Angeles. He and his wife, Penelope, were very much attached to each other, working and traveling together. After she died from cancer of the lung, Spaulding learned of the merit of LJCRF from his friend, Helen Halloran of Escondido. As President of the "Emblem Club" which had made the Foundation the recipient of its donations for the year, she had joined the Foundation's President Club.

Spaulding, a handsome energetic man, visited for one day at the Foundation and had lunch with Lil and I. He was still grieving for "Penny" and described himself as "a very angry man". To our pleasant surprise, we received a check for $100,000 at the Christmas holidays. This donation was repeated a year later. The interest of this money has been used to fund the most promising pilot projects submitted by the scientific staff. Several have produced significant new leads that have been the basis of subsequent successful NIH grant applications.

THE PROGRAM PRINCIPLE AND THE R01 SCIENTIST

A key component in the architecture of the scientific program was the creation of individual research programs. This principle was a major departure from the departmental structure of medical schools. In the latter case, the University allocates laboratory space and a budget to the head of the department. Quite often when a department chairman is replaced, the new head brings in several faculty of his choosing. The existing faculty all experience great insecurity during these transitions except for those who are tenured. University faculty have the opportunity to identify their specific area of research and are under no obligation to interact with other researchers. More often than not, the department chairman is unable to have its members continue at a high level to produce at the cutting edge of the discipline. Then the emphasis switches to teaching and committee work. As a consequence the laboratory space becomes underutilized as ROI grants fail to be renewed. The institution has no effective way to deal with a tenured professor and department chairman who has failed to make his department competitive in research.

At our free-standing Cancer Center, individual scientists were recruited with great attention being paid to their fields of interest in order to match them with the existing ones at the Foundation. Our first putative program leader did not want to review grant applications being submitted by the junior family as he thought this would lessen the independence of the grant writer. Apparently, the desirability for the Institute's prestige to submit only first-class applications was a secondary consideration to him. This unbalanced view of the role of the scientist, the scientific director, and the welfare of the Institute was a negative. His place was taken by Dr. Erkki Ruoslahti who was anxious to advance the field of extracellular matrix interactions. I turned over to him the responsibility of selecting additional staff. One such individual, Dr. Michael Pierschbacher turned out to be a most creative and competent contributor to the extracellular matrix program.

With the NCI approval and funding of this program, we had the credentials to apply for a training grant in order to provide this knowledge of extracellular matrix to post-doctoral students. Dr. Ruoslahti competed successfully for a NCI training grant for the Foundation.

The advantage of the program principle was that if a funded program project failed to remain competitive, the members could regroup and define a different fundamental question to address. There would be no "dead" laboratory space and the challenge to the individual researcher and the group would remain ever fresh and interesting. Also there would be little financial distress to the institution due to major program funds being in jeopardy.

The NCI cancer center philosophy was that the "total should always be greater than the sum of the parts", meaning that evidence of a funded NCI Program Project and Training Grant were the best credentials for a program team effort.

There has always been a question of the "critical mass" and when it can be reached. The "critical mass" at an institution is defined as that number of scientists in a favorable environment which gives the institution a distinctive competitive niche in the world of science. It seemed to us that it was more plausible to achieve a critical mass in a first-class program project, and then to build one program at a time until each achieves a critical mass of both relevant individual and group opportunities. The total of the individual program projects are indeed greater than the sum of its parts.

THE INDUSTRIAL PATRON PROGRAM

The financial structure of the Foundation at the beginning was completely dependent on research grants. A goal was set of securing non-NIH grant funds equal to the research grant total, so that our staff scientists would be dependent on their NIH grants for no more than 50% of their salaries. On the other hand, for scientists to be financially independent of grants would remove from them the obligation to compete with their peers. A consequent drop in performance could be expected.

We visualize the fiscal picture at LJCRF as a stool, resting on three legs; grant support, philanthropy from the community, and industrial support.

The latter was initiated in 1979 as the Industrial Patron program. In return for a donation of $25,000 per annum, the Patron was entitled to visit the Foundation and to talk with its scientists. An invitation to the annual Symposium was included. If the Patron and a scientist found a mutual interest of potential commercial value, a Research and Development agreement would be negotiated. The policy of LJCRF was to share equally with the inventor the funds generated by royalties. The inventor's share would be distributed to him personally and to a research fund for his laboratory.

These policies were instituted in the early 1980s long before biotech-university liaisons were prevalent and accepted.

The first Industrial Patron was the Warner-Lambert Pharmaceutical Corporation with whom I enjoyed good relations from my days at Tufts. A project on the tumor marker, alpha-fetoprotein, was initiated. One of the consistent Industrial Patrons was the Pharmacia Company. It undertook to develop the "sandwich assay" which originated in the Ruoslahti-Engvall laboratories. Others include companies in the U.S., Japan, and Europe; Telios, Monsanto, Hybritech, Genentech, Chugai, Green

Cross, Ono, Mitsubishi, L'Oreal, and Norsk-Hydro.

In 1987, Telios Pharmaceutical Company was established by LJCRF through the combined efforts of Drs. Ruoslahti and Pierschbacher, Theo Heinrichs, Malin Burnham, and T. Knox Bell. It was given an exclusive license to develop and market products arising from the Foundation's patents. In return the Foundation was awarded about 2,500,000 shares and two slots on the Board of Directors of Telios. Subsequently, all other pharmaceutical companies interested in licensing agreements dealt with Telios management. A condition of the licensing agreement with other companies was their becoming Industrial Patrons of LJCRF.

The Trustees of the Foundation agreed that its shares in Telios should provide an endowment fund, a sorely needed credential for the institution.

Industrial Patron policy is turning out to be highly successful and now contributes greatly to the fiscal stability of this institution.

THE NEW BUILDING AND LIBRARY

By 1983, the recruiting of staff was successful to the point that all the laboratory space was completely filled. It was not easy to persuade the Trustees that there were compelling reasons to add laboratory facilities and that a capital campaign would be required. Projections were made on research grant expectations, on further scientist recruitment, on construction costs. Fortunately, Bill Nelson, a developer and financier agreed to be the developer (Nelson had been the negotiator on behalf of the Foundation in arranging the purchase of the Whittaker property on North Torrey Pines Road). He secured three sources of funds; the New England Life Insurance Co., Bank of America, and a group of his private investors.

Malin Burnham had just become Chairman of the Board of

Trustees and had returned from the America Cup races in Newport, R.I. (U.S. lost the Cup to Australia then). He carefully evaluated the plans and gave them his enthusiastic support. With the approval of the Trustees, the administration was authorized to go ahead.

The National Cancer Institute had the authority to make construction grants but the Congress voted only token amounts for the program. We decided to submit an application anyway. The rationale was to provide the space needed to expand the extracellular matrix program for Dr. Ruoslahti and to construct animal facilities that would meet the newer more stringent government regulations. In addition, there was a need for creating shared facilities for protein, carbohydrate and DNA chemistry, to serve the entire staff. We were site-visited by an NCI team of scientists, veterinarians, construction managers, and administrators. The Foundation was approved for a construction grant of $606,900, a huge sum in those days, providing it could be matched from institutional funds. We accepted the challenge.

A fund-raising consultant was recruited, a Mr. Jim Nagle of Newport Beach. Jim was an extravert and an enthusiast. For most of his seventy years, he had been in fund-raising having participated in Eisenhower's presidential campaign. I learned a great deal from him. He placed the highest priority on the Trustees—"the Board! the Board! the Board!" was his constant refrain. "Build the Board!!" He organized the "Capital Fund Cabinet" made up of those trustees who were either or both influential and wealthy. This cabinet met monthly. A Trustee Retreat for one day was held at the University of San Diego, courtesy of Dr. Author Hughes, its President and LJCRF Trustee. From this came a more precise definition of the mission of the Foundation and support for generating industrial participation. A case statement "Commitment to Discovery" was prepared with the help of Nuffer Smith, public relations consultants. The Friends

Auxiliary committed itself to raise money for equipment.

It took two years for the government to fund the $606,900 grant and about the same time for us to raise the matching funds from the Trustees and the community. In the meanwhile, a decision had to be made whether or not to construct a badly-needed library. This would increase the project costs to over $6,000,000. We decided to include the library in the project. It was a wise decision, championed by Trustee Richard B. Huntington;. The library bears his name.

A most disturbing event took place when the buildings were 90% complete. The builders, Equidon Corporation, went bankrupt. Fortunately, Bill Nelson took over the responsibilities of Equidon and completed the buildings.

The great day of dedication of the new building came in February, 1986. The auditorium was crowded. Greetings were extended by representatives of Congressmen, Senators, Mayor, County supervisors, and by the President of the American Association of Cancer Institutes, Dr. Thomas Day. Especially memorable was the keynote speech of the late Dr. Frank Rauscher, Jr., then Senior Vice-President for research at the American Cancer Society. When I drove him to the event, he declared,-"Fishman, you did everything right! Everything!" This was a compliment which I appreciated. In 1992, the new building was named the Walter Fitch III building in recognition of a $1,000,000 gift and his service as a Trustee of LJCRF.

With the new laboratory-administration building, we found ourselves on a higher plateau of credibility. Dr. Michael Pierschbacher set up the protein chemistry lab., Dr. Eva Engvall, the animal facility, Dr. Minoru Fukuda, the carbohydrate chemistry laboratory. These shared facilities created new research capabilities for all the scientific staff. We were able to recruit Dr. Paul Goetinck, who was Director of Molecular Biology at the University of Connecticut at Storrs. He brought with him a small staff and the expertise of the developmental biology of limb development. There was a convergence of interests in the extracellular matrix by both Ruoslahti and Goetinck groups which contributed to the achievement of a "critical mass" in research on the extracellular matrix.

The Huntington library was a key building on the campus. It was built to take advantage of its location amidst the Torrey pine grove—providing outdoor seating and indoor rooms which were illuminated by natural light streaming in through windows set high in the room. It provided a central meeting place for our scientists and a comfortable place to browse through the most recent journals.

HISTORY OF THE ADMINISTRATORS

By the end of the first fiscal year (June 30, 1977), we had a full-time bookkeeper who was supervised once a month by a CPA, Sheldon Derezin, and our first audit was performed by Coopers and Lybrand. Sidney Green was in charge of fiscal matters.

One of our Trustees, Harold Taxel reported to me that the Trustees were uneasy about the fiscal management of the Foundation. Taxel was the publisher of the *La Jolla Light*, a weekly newspaper and had a degree in business administration. Subsequently, he was engaged half-time to supervise Sidney Green and to restructure the business office to meet the concerns of the Trustees.

Taxel was effective and I learned a great deal from him. He told me "The trustees don't like surprises." My practice ever since was to touch base with the Chairman of the Board and Charles Doerr before presenting a fiscal resolution at the Board meeting. This was good advice.

As far as the intricacies of indirect cost rate and fringe benefits, Taxel mastered them quickly. He generated confidence in the management of the Foundation at the frequent NCI site visits we underwent.

We had to deal with the administrative consequences of rapid growth. The Foundation was growing at the rate of 20% per year, the volume of accounting activity rose, shared facilities were being added, new scientific staff was being recruited, and core grant renewal preparations were accelerated. The Foundation was clearly outgrowing the capability of the few administrative staff to serve efficiently. We needed a full-time competent administrator.

Accordingly, we appointed Ken Lasbury, who was an experienced research administrator and had relevant experience at UCSD and Scripps Research Institute. Sally Sullivan, the accounting manager succeeded several accountants who could not keep up with the demands. Sally did and was responsible for computerizing the whole operation. It was successful. A management structure was now in place which has been retained to the present.

Not every project was successful. We were advised to compete for a Cancer Control grant by our consultants. It seemed reasonable that this should focus on the study of tumor markers in a population at high risk for cancer. Dr. Robert Hasterlik, a former Professor of Medicine at the University of Chicago suggested that such a population existed in San Diego by virtue of exposure to asbestos by people who worked in the shipyards during World War II. He was willing to spearhead this effort and so he was appointed an Associate Director for Clinical Affairs. Eventually, a Cancer Control grant application was submitted which was not approved. However, Hasterlik did function well in developing staff policies with the scientists and relating to the community. Subsequently, the major focus of the Foundation then was centered on building up the basic science base.

THE COMMUNITY AND LJCRF

In 1976, I spoke to a colleague who was a successful hematology oncologist in Los Angeles and who administered his own private foundation. I asked him what my chances were of attracting Los Angeles private financial support to the La Jolla Cancer Research Foundation. His answer was that potential donors would first want to know what San Diego thinks of us and how much local support do we attract. This statement convinced me that we had to invest time and effort to become a credible, well-thought of La Jolla institution.

Lil's and my first effort was to host an "open house" at 417 S. Coast Boulevard in the fall of 1977. The scientists each had their own station with posters to illustrate their research and microscopes through which to peer at cancer cells. In the courtyard, a table of refreshments and wine was set up. The Trustees, our neighbors and several friends from Scripps Clinic attended. This was the beginning of the "Friends Auxiliary" of LJCRF under Lil's leadership.

Membership in the Friends was the recruiting goal of a tea at the home of Hilda Hector and of a fashion show at the Women's Club.

The "Dinner under the Stars" was an event enjoyed under a tent in the parking lot, featuring a slide show on China by Dr. Drell. The price of admission was $5, ridiculously low, for an outstanding dinner with all the trimmings. It was well attended.

With events like these the Foundation began to receive favorable attention in the community, although the Cancer League of La Jolla regarded us as unwelcome competition, at first.

The Friends hosted a reception in 1979 to welcome Drs. Erkki Ruoslahti and Eva Engvall to the Foundation. This was attended by the Trustees, staff, and the community. At the opening of the

Torrey Pines facility, the Friends served lunch to all the attendees of the first Foundation Symposium.

The principal focus of the Friends was defined with the necessity to raise $100,000 to match a government grant to fund the purchase of a combination scanning and electron microscope. The Trustees had approved the fund-raising objective but there was a lack of leadership and enthusiasm for the project. However, because of Freddie Deming's enterprise, the Robinson's Department Store at University Town Center agreed to host a fashion show-dinner fund-raiser. This "Robinsons Gala" was attended by many of Freddie's friends and the growing membership of the Friends auxiliary (Richard and Patricia Carlson participated and from then on became staunch supporters of the Foundation). The $25,000 that was the net proceeds of this and other events got the attention of the Trustees who now knew the capital fund campaign was a serious matter. They did respond. Jacques Sherman, who served as President of the Friends, hosted two barbecue fund-raisers at the De Anza resort, at one of which "the Cloggers" dancing group performed.

The next event that Freddie chaired was the "Emerald Affair". This was a shared opportunity between the Inamori jewelry branch of the Kyocera Company. Inamori had perfected a process for making synthetic emeralds and had the ladies of the Friends model them. The Foundation was to receive 10% of the proceeds.

The success of the Robinsons' Gala and the Emerald Affair motivated Patricia Carlson to organize the first "Sentimental Journey". It was a "big band" extravaganza featuring music of the '50's. The star was Patricia's friend and film celebrity Frankie Avalon supported by "The Platters" and "The Coasters". This event was well-attended and raised money towards the "protein sequencer".

A number of small fund-raisers preceded the next Sentimental Journey such as the "Bridge Marathon", a rummage sale and the

"Threepenny Opera". The latter was the first public event at UCSD's new Mandell Weiss Center for Performing Arts and the Friends had the job of filling all the seats for one night at a cost that would cover the UCSD bill and still leave a surplus for the equipment fund. The event was an outstanding success.

"Sentimental Journey II" was chaired again by Patricia Carlson and was held at the Del Mar fairgrounds. This time a Mercedes Convertible donated by the Carlson's was the grand prize of a raffle ticket draw. Altogether $70,000 was raised for the Mass Spectrometer. This amount went a long way to matching a Federal equipment grant of some $100,000. Most important however was the favorable community visibility that was a product of both Sentimental Journeys.

The Friends under Lil's guidance decided to develop a really innovative fund raising event in 1985. This was the "Magical Experience" and it was aided by a master magician, Mr. Stan Gerson. He recruited a number of amateur magicians, taro card readers, psychics, and fortune-tellers who entertained the guests before and during dinner. Afterwards there was presented a professional magician's act on the stage which was followed by dancing. The props, programs, invitations, table centerpieces were all attractive and enhanced the event. Dick Ford was the designer.

It was logical to repeat the event the following year and Magical Experience II was a successful money-raiser. It was used to help purchase the "gene sequencer" apparatus. Junko and Larry Cushman chaired the event.

The Pacesetters was a new auxiliary organized in 1987 by Jo Johnson, Development Manager. Its membership was targeted to younger professionals and business people who would have their own fund-raising goals. After the first membership party, they were able to secure the listing of LJCRF as the beneficiary of a polo match at the San Diego Polo Grounds. Two annual polo events were held with an enthusiastic participation of both young and old. The events raised sufficient funds to buy a Dodge Van for LJCRF. The expectation was that the most committed pacesetters would graduate to membership in President's Council. Also, there was the expectation that this club would facilitate the entry of young executives, professionals and business people into the volunteer activities of the Foundation.

OUR GREAT TRUSTEES

From the beginning, an important question was whether or not the Foundation should have a "rubber-stamp" Board or a working participatory Board. I chose the latter primarily because the Foundation needed the benefit of the intellects, business experience, and community leadership of these individuals. Although a large number of Trustees have come and gone during these past eighteen years and have contributed, there were several whose participation made a big difference to the future of the institution.

WILLIAM DRELL, Ph.D.

Dr. Drell was the President of "Calbiochem" a manufacturer and distributor of biochemical reagent products. I first met Bill Drell when he was a research physiologist at University of California at Los Angeles in 1952. We found research interests in common. He and several others established the California Foundation for Biochemical Research which produced and distributed fine biochemicals. This business increased to the point that it was separated into a for-profit firm "Calbiochem," the Foundation continuing as a separate entity. Its Board of Directors consisted of outstanding California biochemists; Drs. Emil Smith, UCLA; Donald Visser, USC; Eugene Roberts, City of Hope; James Bonner, Cal Tech, and Bill Drell, Calbiochem. Their role was to evaluate applications for summer scholarships from undergraduate students at California research and academic institutions. The funds came from stock transfers from Calbiochem.

Over the years Bill Drell and I developed a warm personal and professional relationship, meeting annually at the Federation of American Societies for Experimental Biology Meetings and in Los Angeles, when I would visit my parents in Elsinore. At times I was able to help Calbiochem in securing biosynthetic enzyme substrates. The original Calbiochem facility looked like a junk yard of plumbing equipment. Large batches of individual amino acids were prepared in second-hand bathtubs, kitchen mixers were employed. There was no front office.

Bill was a dynamic adventurous entrepreneur and in 1959 decided to transfer the business to La Jolla. Mayor Pete Wilson, mayor of San Diego had succeeded in zoning much of the Torrey Pines mesa for research and development firms and for light industry. With the availability of low cost land, Bill established Calbiochem on a 16-acre plot fronting on North Torrey Pines Road. This was to become the "main street" of biomedical research and biotechnology developments in San Diego. Calbiochem was the first company on main street.

Bill Drell was the first scientist we visited in 1975 when Lil and I came to La Jolla. When we inquired whether he would encourage us to relocate to La Jolla, he answered obliquely, "There are a lot of scientists who would like to move to La Jolla, only it is too expensive." However, when we decided to relocate, he gave us his enthusiastic approval.

Bill agreed to become a Trustee but only for a year or two. It turned out to be twelve years instead. It was Bill who suggested Charles D. Doerr, then a Director of Calbiochem, as a candidate for trusteeship. Charlie Doerr was highly regarded in the community for his role as Trustee of the Children's Hospital.

One day in the spring of 1978, I received a most significant phone call from Bill. He asked me if I was prepared to acquire the property across Science Park Road with the help of the California Foundation. This was 4.85 acres fronting Science Park Road on which there were two buildings housing some 20 laboratory areas. It was owned by the Whittaker Corporation in Los Angeles and operated by Microbiological Associates of Maryland. The Facility was designed for contract research on carcinogenic chemicals and viruses and contained safe ventilation to protect personnel. Twenty-five percent of the space was occupied by Microbiological Associates and another 25% was rented to ALS Foundation, Becton-Dickinson Corp., Hansen chemicals. 50% was empty.

The Whittaker Corporation had placed the property on the market for $3,000,000. The California Foundation had found itself with $2,000,000 when it surrendered its stock in Calbiochem to Hoechst Corp. which bought the for-profit firm. The genius of Bill Drell was that he thought of a deal which was a win-win situation for the three parties—LJCRF, California Foundation and the Whittaker Corp. By Whittaker donating the highly appreciated land to LJCRF they benefitted from the tax-exempt status of the donation. That land asset plus the $2,000,000 satisfied the seller and after a series of negotiations the Foundation became owner of the land and master tenant of the two new laboratory buildings. The California Foundation accepted a lease arrangement equivalent to 9.5% return on their $2,000,000. This was a reasonable interest rate at the time.

The lease terms were for twenty years with option to renew. Later, I secured a commitment from the California Foundation to donate the buildings to LJCRF by 1997. As it turned out, the buildings appraised at $2,000,000 were donated on January 1, 1992. The Whittaker gift of the land plus the donated buildings represent the largest gifts to-date to the Foundation.

The support, advice and actions of Bill Drell, Trustee, have made a key difference to the fiscal stability and future of LJCRF.

CHARLES D. DOERR

Erect, tall, grey-haired with a pair of piercing blue eyes, immaculately dressed, Charles D. Doerr's "presence" was commanding. In October 1976, when we were unloading our laboratory equipment from a large moving van in the lane behind the Prospect Avenue Scripps Clinic building, Charlie Doerr greeted us. It seemed that he often took a walk for exercise along that route.

I invited him to visit and he became a frequent visitor. He provided me with names of individuals and organizations who should know about LJCRF. The president of the Chamber of Commerce, Lee Grissom, was one of these.

Charles Doerr was understandably cautious about accepting my invitation for him to become a Trustee. He stated "I need to see evidence of the Foundation's credentials". A couple of months later when we learned that the NCI was funding the Cancer Center planning grant, I presented this evidence of our credentials. He became a Trustee without delay and with a strong commitment.

He had a lifetime experience as an executive in the pharmaceutical industry—McKesson and Robbins—retiring as the firm's treasurer. His voice was always raised against the danger of "red ink" in our fiscal affairs. He also was a leader in fashioning the Foundations by-laws along prudent, responsible lines. He also effectively represented the community at the NCI site visit for the third year of the planning grant.

Most importantly his presence on the Board of Trustees was a significant community credential. Freddie Deming, our star lady Trustee, stated, "I came on the Board because Charlie Doerr was a Trustee."

CAPTAIN ARMISTEAD B. "CHICK" SMITH

Because of my long relationship with Japanese scientists and to a small extent the pharmaceutical industry I was hopeful to recruit the Bank of Tokyo's vice president of the California First Bank, Mr. T. Wakabayashi. He accepted. A short time later, he was succeeded by Yoshi Shibusawa who became an enthusiastic Trustee. When Shibusawa could not attend the Board meetings, he had "Chick" Smith represent him and eventually succeed him when he was transferred to the Los Angeles office.

Captain Smith was an ace Navy fighter pilot who had shot down many "zeros" in combat. After World War II he often attended NATO meetings in Europe and finally became commandant of the Miramar Air Station in San Diego before retirement. California First Bank recruited him as their Vice-President in charge of their Trust Department. His executive ability and his stature in the community led to success of that department at the Bank.

"Chick" knew everyone in San Diego's business, military and lay community. He was recruited to the Trustee Finance Committee where he gave valuable service. He also was instrumental in guiding significant contributions to LJCRF from several private Foundations.

I recall a great year when he was Chairman of the Board. He maintained strong support for the Foundation in all aspects, even in helping at the fundraisers the "Friends" held. As President, it was the first time I experienced the full devotion and undivided commitment of the Chairman of the Board. It was wonderful!

MALIN BURNHAM

A man of priorities and decision is how one would describe Malin Burnham. He was a charming, handsome, tanned, athletic-looking individual with a bunch of hair on his head. When he spoke everyone listened.

He attended a President's Council meeting and became a member soon after. Freddie Deming and Milt Cheverton were Malin's friends and urged him to join. In 1983, he agreed to be a Trustee.

Malin was a fourth generation San Diegan who was president of John Burnham and Company. This successful firm brokered commercial real estate leases and sales plus insurance. He was a leader of the San Diego "establishment".

His hobby was sailing having won a prestigious prize as a teenager. This hobby led to his participation in the America Cup races off Newport for many years and to his leadership in successfully challenging Australia for the Cup they won in 1983. San Diego hosted the 1992 races with Malin at the helm of the Sail America Committee.

By 1983 most of the original Trustees were in their sixth year and there was the desirability of introducing a system of rotation so that Trustees could be brought on board who were best qualified to meet the new and major challenges facing the institution. He sparked the action to review and modify the by-laws to better guide LJCRF.

The biggest Trustee problem was how to replace the Chairman of the Board for the previous six years by an individual who was able and willing to mount a capital campaign to fund the new laboratory building. This was a top priority because the building was essential to accommodate Dr. Ruoslahti's growing research program. If we did not match the government's $606,900 construction grant, the Foundation would be dead in the water and Dr. Ruoslahti would then be planning to accept any one of several good offers from other prestigious institutions.

It should be emphasized that the Chairman and most of the Trustees were capable business and professional people who regarded their role in the Foundation as providing expertise and being unrelated to obligations to make financial contributions. However, the Chairman of the Board, by classic fund-raising principles, is expected to be a major donor. That commitment in turn sets the target for subsequent donors. We needed a new Chairman who would be a major donor.

How does one persuade a Chairman to step aside for the good of the organization? With difficulty! I touched base with Charlie Doerr, Milt Cheverton and Jack Jaynes and they approved my initiative. When I invited the Chairman to step aside but to remain a trustee, he replied, "Bill, I am resigning both as Chairman and Trustee." It took diplomacy and the help of several Trustees to convince the Chairman that resigning as a Trustee would damage the Foundation seriously. He remained as a Trustee.

The one person who was equal to the job expected of Chairman was Malin Burnham. So I asked him. He accepted on the condition that he would serve for three years only. At the end of three years, he did take a year's leave of absence and then returned to the helm until 1994.

To Malin we owe a great deal for his leadership in identifying the important issues, setting them in order of priority and after review and discussion by the Board acting on them. He was a major contributor to the building campaign and helped secure several other major gifts. He made the expertise of John Burnham and Company available to the Foundation's administration. This was particularly valuable in arranging the best terms for financing the construction of the new building. Finally, Malin did attract a number of his friends to the Board who were helpful in monitoring the progress of the construction, e.g. Dean Dunphy and Hal Sadler. Malin supported all of the Foundation's fundraisers either by an underwriting contribution or by filling one or two tables.

The period of the '80s in San Diego was marked by the birth of biotechnology companies whose role model was "Hybritech" which successfully commercialized monoclonal antibody diagnostic test kits. Incidentally, Hybritech's first facility was leased from the Foundation.

Malin was convinced that it was essential to accelerate the transfer of basic research findings to pharmaceutical products benefitting patients. This would provide a clearer community understanding of the role of the Foundation in therapy of patients and also, if successful, could be a third source of income—grants and gifts being the first two. His recommendation was to hire a broker who would seek to interest venture capitalists in the Foundations discoveries.

It seemed to me that Dr. Ruoslahti should lead this effort because as the next President and as Scientific Director and as the major inventor, he would have to accept or not accept the expected proposals. It would eliminate a "middle man" who would have to be educated on the scientific merit of the discoveries. One day, Erkki confessed to me that he was bored. I immediately offered him the challenge of creating the commercial arm of the Foundation to his liking. He accepted happily.

With the creation of the Telios Pharmaceutical Company, Malin Burnham and Erkki Ruoslahti became members of the Telios Board of Directors to represent the interests of the Foundation. The Foundation's stake was some 2,500,000 shares which was balanced by a $3,000,000 investment by the investors. The Foundation was to receive royalty income when products came to market. Dr. Michael Pierschbacher, a co-inventor of the RGD-fibronectin cell adhesion domain, became Director of Research at Telios. Dr. Theo Heinrichs of Hambrecht and Qvist, a San Francisco firm, was chief executive officer and Chairman of the Board of Directors. Later Dr. Robert Erickson became President and CEO.

What was manifestly clear in Burnham's history with the Foundation was that he did not shrink from meeting challenges which at first sight were overwhelming, providing the challenge was of first priority. The Foundation will always be indebted for his leadership.

THE HONORABLE WILL HIPPEN, JR.

In 1980, I and Dr. Hirai arranged a US-Japan conference centered on oncodevelopmental biology to be held at the Del Coronado Hotel in December. It was necessary to recruit a speaker who would address the participants after the Conference dinner: someone who could relate to both Japanese and American cultures. I asked Mr. Shibusawa of the California First Bank whom he would recommend. He gave me the name of the Honorary Consul General for Japan at San Diego—Mr. Will Hippen, Jr. Will accepted and gave a very fine address.

Later when we had lunch together in the Sky Room of the La Valencia, I learned that we shared a number of experiences and interests. Born on the prairie in Oklahoma, he had finished two years of medical school before he enlisted in the merchant marine during World War II and served in the Pacific. His twin brother, Robert received his M.D. and practiced Urology in San Diego.

Will met a widow, Mary Summerlin, and they were married. But Mary Summerlin was no ordinary woman. She had become a professional cytotechnologist having trained at the Sloan-Kettering Institute in New York. She established a cytotechnology training program at Sharp Hospital in San Diego and endowed it with a substantial sum of money before she died.

Because of our mutual interest in oncology and in Japan-US relations, it was natural to invite Will Hippen to join the Board of Trustees. He accepted with enthusiasm and became Chairman of President's Council. It flourished under his leadership.

A glimpse of his humanity was evident when I and Malin

Burnham invited him to contribute to the capital campaign. We suggested the sum of $50,000. He did not blink but asked if his donation could memorialize his friend, Dr. Michael J. Feeney, who was dying from prostatic cancer. The gift was pledged over five years, the last two of which came from Will Hippen's estate as inoperable intestinal cancer shortened his life.

EUGENE ROBERTS, Ph.D.

Dr. Roberts and his family met the Fishmans in the summer of 1951 in Bar Harbor, Maine. Eugene was studying amino acid patterns in tumors of different strains of inbred mice and I was investigating the response to androgens and estrogens of ß-glucuronidase in various tissues of a number of strains of inbred mice. The Jackson Laboratory was a world center for the propagation of pedigreed mice which they supplied to investigators all over the world.

Next, in 1952, we both attended an International Congress of Biochemistry in Paris. The most memorable event was our visit with Raoul Dufy previously described. For years afterwards whenever I was in Los Angeles, we would meet in Duarte at the City of Hope. Eugene's interest for many years was amino acid metabolism in cancer but when he discovered gamma-aminobutyric acid, a neurotransmitter, his interest was then directed to the neurosciences.

Eugene's membership at City of Hope helped the Foundation. Drs. Ruoslahti and Engvall were his colleagues at City of Hope and they asked his advice on moving to the La Jolla Cancer Research Foundation and his opinion of Fishman. Obviously they were satisfied with the answers.

Similarly Eugene's being a Director of the California Foundation for Biochemical Research was similarly helpful. He was a strong articulate supporter of Bill Drell's plan to invest $2,000,000 in the buildings of LJCRF and an enthusiastic admirer of what had been accomplished at the Foundation.

His role in LJCRF became even more significant as a long time member of its Board of Scientific Advisors and culminated in his election to the Board of Trustees in 1990. His influence with the California Foundation was important in their making the decision to donate their two buildings to LJCRF in 1992 rather than 1997.

WALTER FITCH III

Walter Fitch came into the Foundation Board of Trustees almost by osmosis. He attended the "Magical Experience" fund-raisers and found his enjoyment was shared by Freddie Deming and Lee Weston. In addition, he learned more about the Foundation from his friend Chick Smith.

Walter comes from an established family in Coronado, an island next to San Diego. He was a pilot with Pan Am from 1941-51. He is proud of the pioneering done by Pan Am.

Subsequently he became the founder and Chairman of the Board of Texas Oil and Gas. In 1984, it was acquired by U.S. Steel.

Walter projects a warm charming personality with a sense of humor which lights up his blue eyes to twinkling intensity. In San Diego he is widely respected for his generous philanthropy. The Foundation has received $1,000,000 towards its Project 2000 capital campaign. This gift has been recognized by naming the 32,000 sq. ft. building, completed in 1985, as the Walter Fitch III building.

He remains very active and supportive of the President, the Trustees and the staff of LJCRF.

RICHARD B. HUNTINGTON

Dick Huntington is widely perceived to be a vigorous thoughtful and warm individual. In San Diego he is respected for his successes in the construction industry and its financing. He has served as a Director of the La Jolla Bank and Trust and now as a Director of the Scripps Bank. His community philanthropies have centered on the Bishops School and the La Jolla Cancer Research Foundation. In the latter institution, he has underwritten the Richard B. Huntington Library. It serves the entire scientific community at the Foundation.

CHAPTER 17

THE TRANSITION OF LEADERSHIP

In the early years of the Foundation, a perennial question which Trustees asked was, "What happens to the Foundation if Fishman gets hit by a truck?" This stimulated the formulation of a plan for this contingency. One part was to take out a "key man" insurance policy for $1,000,000 which would provide funds to find and support the new President. Another aspect was to define a "search committee" whose responsibility it would be to search for the best replacement possible. One qualification was put forward—that the President be either an active scientist or a senior person with a strong science background. This was believed necessary because the executive had to have an operational understanding of what makes scientists tick and of how to maintain an environment conducive to the best science.

With Dr. Ruoslahti serving as the Scientific Director there was reason to believe that the scientific program would not be seriously damaged by the loss of the President. The science would continue.

As the years went by, it became clear to me that Dr. Ruoslahti was demonstrating considerable administrative abilities and that his ambition was to succeed me and "take a crack" at leading the Foundation into the future. Since he was heading a team of scientists who were making history in the new field of adhesive proteins and integrins, it was in the best interest of LJCRF to provide him every opportunity to advance and to keep open for him the option of the succession to the Presidency.

The big question now was "when". The Trustees would have had no objection if I stayed on as President to the end of my days.

However, I doubted whether Erkki, who was receiving marvellous offers for Department Chairs in first-rate universities, would wait indefinitely for his opportunity. I made the decision publicly in 1987 to seek "emeritus" status at age seventy-five which would be March 2, 1989. It was also made clear that Dr. Ruoslahti was the heir-apparent and this view was accepted by the Trustees.

Erkki attached one condition to the succession plan—that he could have the Administrator and Grants Manager of his own choosing.

So from 1987 on, all significant personnel hirings required Erkki's approval so that by 1989 he would have his own crew on board. Also, Erkki prepared a ten-year plan for the Foundation which expressed his goal of expanding the size, scope, and research program three-fold.

THE NEW ADMINISTRATOR

The Foundation engaged Korn Ferry, an executive search firm to find candidates for the position of Administrator. The "headhunters" came up with two candidates who were scientists and administrators. The one Erkki chose was Dr. Douglas Armstrong from the Pharmacology Department of the University of California at San Francisco.

Doug stood about six feet five inches with a handsome unwrinkled baby face from which a pair of steel blue eyes shone. He had a winning personality and received widespread enthusiastic approval. It became clear that he was extremely ambitious but was injecting a philosophy of micro-managing into every single activity in the administration. When Sally Sullivan who ran the accounting department efficiently for years didn't satisfy him with "creative financing" proposals, he hired an individual to whom Sally was to report—a demotion. She left immediately for an excellent position at Scripps Memorial

Hospital. He had the Personnel Manager monitor the comings and goings of the Foundation photographer. He told all the personnel they could be replaced—an expression of intimidation which was an entirely new tone to LJCRF.

Doug was certain that he could bring in the private contributions and Foundation grants in the millions as Erkki's plan demanded. In meetings with development officers in our neighboring institutions, he was convinced that the "Friends Auxiliary" was a cost ineffective way to raise money. Accordingly, Doug designed a set of regulatory controls over the volunteers that the "Friends" found unacceptable. Subsequently, they voted to disband their organization. The fund-raising efforts of Doug were complete failures as it turned out.

THE TRANSITION

As far as achievements in the grant arena were concerned, all the institutional grants were renewed by July 1, 1989 for five years. These included the Core Grant, Dr. Ruoslahti's program project, Dr. Goetinck's program project and two teaching grants for post-docs. These credentials would keep the Foundation going for five years and represented the prestige of the institution.

The Trustees created an Ad Hoc Leadership Transition Committee to define conditions for Dr. and Mrs. Fishman to continue to serve the Foundation and other details such as relocation of offices and secretarial staff. By virtue of Dr. Fishman serving on the Core Grant Renewal Application as Deputy Director, he was compensated as a consultant at half his salary. Mrs. Fishman was also offered a consultantship in the office of the President Emeritus. Finally, the Trustees voted Emeritus status and made Dr. Fishman a Life Trustee. In addition, a Chair to be named the William H. Fishman Chair was committed. A portrait of Bill and Lil Fishman was commissioned and the Auditorium was named the Fishman Auditorium.

Two Tribute events were held to honor the Fishmans. On February 1 to 3, 1989, Dr. José L. Millán organized a Symposium on Alkaline Phosphatases which was attended by scientists from U.K., Belgium, Russia, Japan, Canada and the U.S. Later an entire issue (46) of *Clinica Chimica Acta* included significant papers of the Symposium. Next on March 1 under the Chair of Elsie Weston, a formal "Tribute to the Fishmans" dinner was held at the Marriott Hotel. It was attended by a cross-section of the citizenry of San Diego, an indication of the roots LJCRF had made in the community.

The transition was now complete. Dr. Erkki Ruoslahti became the second president of the La Jolla Cancer Research Foundation.

CHAPTER 18

TECHNOLOGY TRANSFER-TELIOS PHARMACEUTICAL CO.

From the time the Foundation was founded, there was the commitment to make it much less dependent on Federal funding of research. The goal was to provide sufficient non-government support to cover half the salary of each Principal Investigator. There were two reasonable sources we identified: one was contributions from individual donors and grants from Foundations, the other was industrial support.

We established the Industrial Patron Program in 1977 described in Chapter 16.

When Drs. Ruoslahti and Engvall developed the two-site "sandwich" assay for alpha-fetoprotein, they contacted Dr. Lundquist at Pharmacia in Uppsala, Sweden. Subsequently, Pharmacia became the second Industrial Patron.

When I was at Tufts, I met a representative of the Monsanto Company who was the Director of their "New Enterprises" division. By 1980, I contacted him and accepted an invitation to explain the mission of the La Jolla Cancer Research Foundation to a few key executives. Apparently they found it persuasive and Monsanto joined the Industrial Patrons.

Through an introduction by Dr. Hirai, I met Dr. R. Naito the President of the Green Cross Corporation in Osaka. He visited the Foundation along with the President, Dr. Tom Drees, of the Green Cross affiliate, the Alpha-Therapeutic Corp. Subsequently, the Green Cross Corporation became an Industrial Patron.

A spurt in growth of membership took place as a result of the establishment of the Telios Pharmaceutical Company. They required that their major investors from the pharmaceutical world become members of the Industrial Patron Club. As a result, the following firms joined: Telios, Ono Pharmaceutical, Norsk-Hydro, Matsushita, and Genentech.

With the Industrial Patron Program, the administration and the staff became better informed as to its potential for supporting research, both short term and long term. It also led to a sense of partnership whereby everyone wins. The Foundation secured the patents on the discoveries of its staff and established generous terms for the distribution of royalty income. Thus, 50% would go to the inventor and his laboratory in a ratio of two to one and 50% would be the Foundation's share. Ultimately, royalty income was expected to become substantial and could help meet whose costs which could not be met by government grants.

TECHNOLOGY TRANSFER

By 1986, it had become clear that patents which the Foundation held had potential utility in generating products of importance at the bedside. Our Chairman of the Board was very enthusiastic to demonstrate that the basic research at LJCRF was benefitting humanity. I was regularly prodded to find a broker who would market the Foundation's discoveries.

By this time, I had observed that Dr. Ruoslahti had a talent of communicating and dealing with businessmen in the Pharmaceutical arena. Also, no matter who I found as the broker, Dr. Ruoslahti as Scientific Director and inventor would be making the decisions. I asked him to take on the responsibility of technology transfer completely and that I would support him. He agreed happily. This was another milestone in the history of LJCRF.

THE TELIOS PHARMACEUTICAL COMPANY

Erkki very quickly began to contact venture capital companies and to invite their interest in creating a for-profit company that would have responsibility for identifying commercially feasible products generated by the discoveries at the Foundation and to bring them to market. Through Knox Bell, Foundation counsel, Dr. Theo Heinrichs of the San Francisco Venture Capital firm of Hambrecht and Quist was introduced to Dr. Ruoslahti. The chemistry was right.

At this time, there was considerable debate in the academic community as to the degree of propriety which should be operating in the role in industry of academic scientists of a non-profit research institution. Questions of conflict of interest, interference in the free dissemination of research results, etc. were raised.

It was decided that the firm be completely independent of the Foundation with its own President, CEO, and Board of Directors. The Foundation would be assigned half the original shares in exchange for the technology while the venture firms invested $3,000,000 for the "start-up". Two representatives of the Foundation were assigned seats on the Board of Directors. The firm would take over the manufacture and distribution of monoclonal antibodies and extracellular matrix products which were in demand. Finally, Telios became a most significant Industrial Patron in 1987.

Five years later, the Telios Pharmaceutical Company is housed in a new 65,000 sq. ft. building in the "Golden Triangle" area of San Diego with some 150 employees. The Golden Triangle is the area included between routes I-5 and 805 as they merge together into I-5 North. The facility is equipped with the most modern improvements—clean air rooms, hot pure distilled water circulation, protein chemistry synthesis, super quality control of the total environment.

Three products are in various stages of manufacture and clinical trials. An application to the FDA (Food and Drug Administration) has been submitted for "Argidine Healing Gel", a product which promotes wound-healing. Another is a preparation which is effective against "dry eye", a condition of inadequate supply of tears. A most interesting application is the use of a cyclic RGD peptide which disaggregates platelet clumps to aid the dissolution of blood clots in the coronary arteries.

CHAPTER 19

ERKKI RUOSLAHTI - SECOND PRESIDENT OF LJCRF, 1989-

Erkki Ruoslahti was born in Finland on the 16th of February, 1940 in the eastern province of Karelia. His father was a builder of power plants and other industries in Finland, providing a background which benefitted Erkki in his later handling of financial and other transactions with the pharmaceutical industry.

He received the M.D. degree in 1965 from the University of Helsinki and then did a thesis for the Doctorate of Immunology in the Department of Serology and Bacteriology. There he worked as a Research and Teaching Assistant, becoming head of the Blood Group Department at the State Serum Institute from 1966 to 1968.

A most significant event was the next three years he spent at the California Institute of Technology in Pasadena as an NIH Research fellow in the laboratory of Dr. William Brewer. He absorbed not only state of the art knowledge of techniques and principles of immunochemistry but the culture of American science and its emphasis on competition and the peer review process.

He returned to the University of Helsinki and in 1975, at the age of thirty-five, he was appointed Professor of Bacteriology and Serology at the University of Turku. Six months later he was accepted as a visiting scientist at the National Cancer Institute in William Terry's laboratory in Washington (54).

This last experience coupled with his stay at Cal Tech convinced Ruoslahti that to advance his scientific career he should find an opportunity in the United States. It was only a short time later before Dr. Charles Todd of the City of Hope in Duarte,

California offered him a position of Senior Research Scientist. It was accepted and only eight months later he was promoted to the position of Director of Immunobiology in the Department of Immunology.

This move was significant also for another reason. Dr. Eva Engvall who had received her Ph.D. in Immunology at the University of Stockholm in 1975 became an EMBO post-doctoral fellow in the Department of Serology and Bacteriology at the University of Helsinki. There she met Erkki and a life-long partnership in life and science began at that moment. She joined Erkki at the City of Hope.

Drs. Ruoslahti and Engvall were both highly regarded in the field of oncodevelopmental biology for their work on the chemistry and biology of alpha-fetoprotein (55), pregnancy-specific ß-globulin (56) and CEA (57). They had initiated a major effort to isolate and evaluate the cell attachment site of fibronectin, an adhesive protein. The problem at City of Hope was that Dr. Todd placed a low priority on this initiative relative to his own interest in CEA. This led to frustration of such a degree that in 1979, the team of Ruoslahti and Engvall began to search for their next opportunity.

They had attended the 1976 San Diego meeting of the oncodevelopmental biologists and became aware of the potential the field offered and the role of its prime organizer in the U.S.

In 1978, I defined an essential need for a brilliant young scientist, identified as an oncodevelopmental biologist to fill the number two position at the Foundation. On reviewing the list of attendees at the San Diego 1976 meeting, two names stood out. One was Dr. Stuart Sell of the Department of Pathology at UCSD and the other was Dr. Ruoslahti.

Dr. Sell and I had a good professional relationship; each of us with a different but complementary research interest. He was highly regarded for his research on alpha-fetoprotein and with his expertise in immunology and pathology he could greatly fortify the Foundation's credibility and relevance to human cancer. He did contribute a component to the Program Project application I submitted in September 1976 and he was the co-editor of *Oncodevelopmental Gene Expression*. However, he believed he was better off in a secure tenured professorship at UCSD.

Dr. Ruoslahti, on the other hand, had as his highest priority the opportunity to pursue his research objectives with all his vigor but without control of his career or opportunity by scientist administrators or by a pre-occupation with tenure. He had great confidence in his ability to compete successfully for NIH grants. All he needed was sufficient laboratory space and unqualified support by the President. This I could and did provide.

Dr. Engvall was a first class scientist in her own right. She and Dr. Perlmann at the University of Stockholm were amongst the first to report the ELISA technology (58) which today is the most widely employed analytical procedure used in the hospital clinical laboratory for measuring a host of antigenic proteins and other biological materials. Her sure instincts for isolating pure proteins from biological sources led to her introducing Sepharose-collagen columns as a means of rescuing fibronectin from such sources. After washing off impurities, the fibronectin could be recovered from the column in pure condition (59).

I recall that Dr. Ruoslahti transported such a column in his car the day he arrived in La Jolla and transferred it to the cold room. Not a minute was lost in the transfer of their research from City of Hope to the Foundation.

Dr. Ruoslahti had committed himself to put together a Program Project grant application by October 1. It was essential for the Foundation to demonstrate that its investigators could relate their work to a worthwhile scientific goal which as individuals they were not capable of achieving. In short order, we recruited Dr. Charles Birdwell from the Salk Institute who attracted an excellent electron microscopist, George Klier to operate the electron microscope facility and Dr. Eileen Adamson, a developmental biologist from Oxford University. Erkki confessed to me that his stomach would be knotted from the stress of the challenge of putting together the Program Project. It was site-visited by a peer review committee, received a high score, and was funded for three years. It continues on a five year funding cycle.

This success supported the first Core Grant application which was site visited and funded by the NCI.

Dr. Michael Pierschbacher was the first postdoctoral student from La Jolla to work with Dr. Ruoslahti. He came from Dr. Katz's laboratory at Scripps Clinic. Dr. Katz was rumored to have said that Michael had no future in scientific research. How wrong he was!

With the availability of pure fibronectin, Pierschbacher and Ruoslahti proceeded to split it into fragments and in short order they were able to identify a collagen-binding domain and a cell attachment domain (60). Pierschbacher then flew to Uppsala, Sweden, where he established the amino acid sequence of these domains under the guidance of Per Petersen. On his return, it was possible to narrow the cell attachment domain to a sequence of three amino acids, arginine, glycine, and aspartic acid. Translated into the single letter amino acid code, this is the RGD sequence.

This discovery has stimulated a tremendous amount of research in the fields of oncology and developmental biology and has earned for Dr. Ruoslahti and his colleagues great recognition. It also provided a new focus and direction of much of the Foundation research which was to follow.

EPILOGUE

In my opinion, an institute either has or does not have a soul. It is not easy to define an institute's soul but it is not difficult at all to recognize the absence of soul.

In too many cases, scientists on the faculty of Universities find that they become victims of academic knifing and cruelty. This can happen to individuals whose research is competitive, whose teaching is first-class and whose collegiality and committee work are more than satisfactory.

On the other hand, a faculty member can be described as "an excellent scientist but a rotten human being." When such an individual achieves adminstrative power, the department becomes the possession of the chairman and is often used to promote the chairman's career at the expense of the independence of the department members. Anyone who does not play ball with the boss runs the risk of a negative recommendation for tenure.

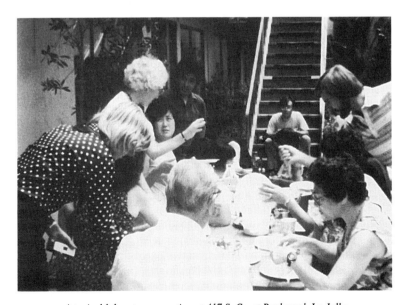

A typical laboratory reception at 417 S. Coast Boulevard, La Jolla

At the La Jolla Cancer Research Foundation, Lil and I had created a family atmosphere which was inclusive. New staff members were publicly welcomed. Visitors from abroad were helped. Foundation picnics, Thanksgiving and Christmas parties brought the individual families together.

With the program infrastructure, no individual could become a department chairman in the University sense. This means that each scientist has the same rights, privileges and responsibilities provided they pass peer review of their grant applications at the National Institutes of Health. No one individual could torpedo a promotion because of the democratic structure of our promotion process.

Then there are the intangibles which contribute to the soul of the institute. For example, the buildings are positioned in a grove of rare Torrey Pine trees which tower 80 to 100 feet over the grounds. The grounds are covered with vinca and in the spring a number of flowering trees burst into bloom. Every year migrating Monarch butterflies make a rest stop on the grounds as do many species of birds and animals.

Many a staff member has said that the environment at the Foundation is so attractive and tranquil that it helps them considerably. They are not tired at the end of the day.

Finally, the institute has been adopted by the community since its creation.

This community interest and support as evidenced by an outstanding Board of Trustees plus the President's leadership which is positive and committed plus the happiness of the staff which is provided the very best research opportunities all combine to give LJCRF its identity and humanity.

Finally, additional recognition to Dr. Fishman in the form of the 1993 ISOBM Abbott Award came at the 21st meeting of the International Society for Oncodevelopmental Biology which was held in Jerusalem on November 8 (61). Earlier in 1983, Umeå

University in Sweden conferred an honorary M.D. degree upon Dr. Fishman in recognition of the value of his laboratory research to Medicine.

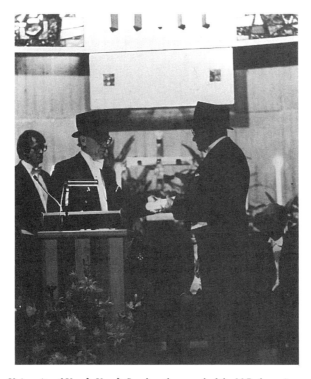

At the University of Umeå, Umeå, Sweden, the award of the M.D. honoris causae to Dr. William H. Fishman, Ph.D. in recognition of his contributions to medicine, 1983

APPENDIX A

ARTICLES OF INCORPORATION - LA JOLLA CANCER RESEARCH FOUNDATION

I - NAME
The name of this Corporation is:
LA JOLLA CANCER RESEARCH FOUNDATION.

II - PURPOSE
The purposes for which this Corporation is formed are:

(a) The specific and primary purpose for which this Corporation is formed is to establish, own and operate an interdisciplinary Center for Onco-Developmental Sciences, which Center will perform fundamental basic and clinical research to advance knowledge in the interrelated sciences of oncology and of developmental biology, commonly known as "onco-developmental sciences". The center's goal is to achieve a more precise understanding of the nature and etiology of cancer and other developmental diseases and disorders so that the Center can originate and carry out demonstrations of advanced techniques for diagnosis, treatment and rehabilitation for the benefit of the patient with cancer and other developmental diseases and anomalies; including, without limitation, programs of research, education, lectures, conferences, training, epidemiology, publication and community participation. The Corporation shall have the power to do all necessary or incidental acts in the furtherance of its specific and primary purpose.

(b) The Corporation shall have all the general purposes and powers conferred on non profit corporations under the laws of California, as such laws exist from time to time, including without limitation, the general purposes and powers:

(1) To solicit, collect, receive, acquire, hold and invest money and property, both real and personal, received by gift, contribution, bequest, devise, or otherwise; to sell and convert property, both real and personal, into cash; and to use the funds of this Corporation and the proceeds, income, rents, issues and profits derived from any property of this Corporation for any of the purposes for which this corporation is formed.

(2) To purchase or otherwise acquire, own, hold, sell, assign, transfer or otherwise dispose of, mortgage, pledge or otherwise hypothecate or encumber, and to deal in and with shares, bonds, notes, debentures, or other securities or evidences of indebtedness of any person, firm, corporation or association and, while the owner or holder thereof, to exercise all rights, powers and privileges of ownership.

(3) To purchase, lease or otherwise acquire, own, hold, use, sell, exchange, assign, convey, lease or otherwise dispose of and mortgage or otherwise hypothecate or encumber real or personal property.

(4) To invest and reinvest its funds in such stock, common or preferred, bonds, debentures, mortgages, or in such other securities and property as its board of directors shall deem advisable, subject to the limitations and conditions contained in any bequest, devise, grant, or gift, provided such limitations and conditions are not in conflict with any provision of the Internal Revenue Code of 1954, as amended, and its regulations as they now exist or as they may hereafter be amended.

(5) To borrow money, incur indebtedness and to secure the repayment of the same by mortgage, pledge, deed of trust, or other hypothecation of property, both real and personal.

(6) To carry into effect any one or more of the objects and purposes hereinabove set forth and to that end to do any one or more of the acts and things aforesaid, and likewise any and all acts or things necessary or incidental thereto; and, in conducting or carrying on its activities, and for the purpose of promoting or furthering any one or more of its said objects or purposes, to exercise any or all of the powers hereinabove set forth in this Article, and any other or additional power now or hereafter authorized by law, either alone or in conjunction with others, as principal, agent, partner, joint venturer, share holder, member, contractor, or otherwise; provided, however, that this Corporation shall not, except to an insubstantial degree, engage in any activities or exercise any powers that are not in furtherance of the primary purpose of this Corporation.

(c) Notwithstanding any other provision of these Articles of Incorporation, this Corporation shall not have the power to, and shall not, do any act or conduct any activity, plan, scheme, design, or course of conduct which in any way conflicts with the following specific prohibitions:

1. No part of the net earnings of the Corporation shall inure to the benefit of any member, trustee, officer or private person.

2. No substantial part of the activities of the Corporation shall consist of the carrying on of propaganda, or otherwise attempting, to influence legislation.

3. The Corporation shall not, either directly or indirectly, participate in, or intervene in (including the publishing or distributing of statements), any political campaign on behalf of or in opposition to any candidate for public office.

4. The property of the Corporation must be used exclusively for

charitable, scientific, and educational purposes meeting the requirements of Section 214 of the California Revenue and Taxation Code.

5.   The property of the Corporation shall not be used or operated so as to benefit any officer, trustee, member, employee, contributor, or any other person, through the distribution of profits, payment of excessive charges or compensation, or the more advantageous pursuit of their business or profession to the exclusion of other qualified persons.

6.   The property of the Corporation shall not be used by the trustees, officers, members, employees, contributors or other persons for fraternal or lodge purposes, or for social club purposes, except where such use is clearly incidental to the Corporation's primary charitable, scientific, or educational purposes.

III - NONPROFIT ORGANIZATION
This Corporation is organized for nonprofit purposes pursuant to the General Nonprofit Corporation Law of the State of California. This Corporation does not contemplate pecuniary gain or profit to the members thereof.

IV - PRINCIPAL OFFICE
The County in this State where the principal office for the transaction of the business of this Corporation is located in San Diego County.

V - TRUSTEES
The names and addresses of the persons who are to act in the capacity of Trustees until the selection of their successors are:

NAMES	ADDRESSES
T. Knox Bell	2100 Union Bank BuildingSan Diego, California 92101
Kenneth G. Coveney	2100 Union Bank BuildingSan Diego, California 92101
Joan K. Greenwood	2100 Union Bank BuildingSan Diego, California 92101

The number of Trustees shall be three (3) until such number shall be changed by an amendment to these Articles or by a Bylaw duly adopted by the members. The qualifications, term and duties of Trustees shall be as stated in the Bylaws.

VI - MEMBERS
The authorized number and qualifications of members of the Corporation, the different classes of membership, if any, the property, voting and other rights and privileges of members, and their liability for dues and assessments and the method of collection thereof, shall be as set forth in the Bylaws.

VII - DEDICATION AND DISSOLUTION

The property, assets, profits and net income of this Corporation are irrevocably dedicated to charitable, scientific, and educational purposes meeting the requirements of Section 214 of the California Revenue and Taxation Code, and no part of the net income or assets of this organization shall ever inure to the benefit of any trustee, officer, member, or private person. On the dissolution or winding up of this Corporation, its assets remaining after payment of, or provision made for the payment of, all debts and liabilities of this Corporation shall be distributed to a nonprofit fund, foundation or corporation which is organized and operated exclusively for charitable, scientific and educational purposes meeting the requirements of Section 214 of the California Revenue and Taxation Code, and which has established its tax-exempt status under Section 501 (c) (3) of the Internal Revenue Code of 1954, as amended. If such assets are not so disposed of by the Trustees of this Corporation, such assets shall be disposed of in such a manner as may be directed by decree of the Superior Court of the county in which the corporation has its principal office on petition therefor by the Attorney General or by any person concerned in the liquidation in a proceeding to which the Attorney General is a party.

IN WITNESS WHEREOF, the undersigned, being the persons hereinabove named as the first directors, have executed these Articles of Incorporation, this 7th day of July, 1976.

Signed:
T. Knox Bell
Kenneth G. Coveney
Joan K. GreenwoodB

APPENDIX B

ROSTER OF ADMINISTRATION, STAFF, AND TRUSTEES (1994)

ADMINISTRATIVE STAFF

Erkki Ruoslahti, M.D.
President & Chief Executive Officer

Louis R. Coffman
Vice President, Chief Administrative Officer

Nancy J. Beddingfield
Executive Assistant to the President
Secretary, LJCRF

Jennifer East
Purchasing Manager

Jean Freiser
Sponsored Programs Manager

Paula Kamphaus
Information Systems Manager

Sherri Marinovich
Human Resources Director

Stephen A. Moglia
Controller

Keith Short
Chief Financial Officer

Carl W. Crader
Physical Plant Manager

Rhonda H. Jenkins
Animal Resources Manager

John W. Knight
DNA Facility Manager

Muizz Hasham
Biomedical Communications Manager

Khanh T. Nguyen
Protein Chemistry Manager

Taras T. Gach
Vice President, Resource Programs

Pandi Veerapandian
Scientific Computer Center Manager

Jacqueline Avis
Transgenic Mouse Facility Manager

Larry Adelman
Occupational Health & Safety Manager

Kathryn Ely, Ph.D.
Staff Scientist & Community Scientific Liaison

Crystal Herndon
Executive Assistant to the Chief Administrative Officer

SCIENTIFIC STAFF

Erkki Ruoslahti, M.D.
Scientific Director

Robert G. Oshima, Ph.D.
Associate Scientific Director

Senior Staff Scientists
Eileen D. Adamson, Ph.D.
Eva S. Engvall, Ph.D.
Hudson H. Freeze, Ph.D.
Michiko N. Fukuda, Ph.D.
Minoru Fukuda, Ph.D.
Terumi Kohwi-Shigematsu, Ph.D.
José Luis Millán, Ph.D.
Magnus Pfahl, Ph.D.
William B. Stallcup, Ph.D.

Staff Scientists
Michael D. Pierschbacher,
Ph.D. (adjunct appointment)
Adrienne Brian, Ph.D.
Gregg L. Duester, Ph.D.
Kathryn R. Ely, Ph.D.
Richard A. Maki, Ph.D.
Joseph Parello, Ph.D.
Elena Pasquale, Ph.D.
Barbel E. Ranscht, Ph.D.
John C. Reed, M.D., Ph.D.

Assistant Staff Scientists
Nuria Estel Assa-Munt, Ph.D.
Hélène Baribault, Ph.D.
Steven Frisch, Ph.D.
Craig Hauser, Ph.D.
Shi Huang, Ph.D.
Yoshinori Kohwi, Ph.D.
Wanda F. Reynolds, Ph.D.
Yu Yamaguchi, M.D., Ph.D.
Xiaokun Zhang, Ph.D.

Visiting Scientists
Sara Szuchet

Postdoc's
Hwee Luan Ang
Ayse Batova
Erik Berglund
Ger Boonen
Michael Burg
Kyle Chan
Lisa Dukhang Chong
Robert James Connor
Ian deBelle
Louise Deltour
Craig Dickinson
Karen Dolter
James Etchison
Fang Fang
Andrea Noemi Fanjul
Beatriz Ferreiro
Barbara Fredette
Kathryn Grako
Gerhart A. Graupner
Motoi Hanada
Masayoshi Harigai
Terry F. Hayamizu
John Hirai
Marie-Claude Hofmann
Jocelyn Holash
Renate Kain

Shinya Kaname
Shami Kanekar
Nicholas Kenney
Shinichi Kitada
Erkki Koivunen
Erich Koller
Stanislaw Krajewski
Nathalie LaVista
Mi-Ock Lee
Yin Li
Yi Liu
Angela Lombardo
Xian Ping Lu
Deidre MacKenna
Scott R. McKercher
Darshini Mehta
Toshiyuki Miyashita
Alex O. Morla
Nickolay Neznanov
Chao-Zhou Ni
Gertraud Orend
Krishnasamy Panneerselvam
Timo Pikkarainen
Frederic Pio
Antje Portner
Kodandapani Ramadurgam
Katherine Rhodes
Laura Richardson
Fransoise Roquet
Gilles Salbert
Takaaki Sato
Gang Shao
Motoyuki Shimonaka
David Skrincosky
Chandrasen Soans
Geetha Srikrishna
George Steele-Perkins
Shinichi Takayama
Shigeru Tsuboi
Ichiro Ueno
Bingcheng Wang
Yilong Wang
Hong-Gang Wang
Ken Watanabe
Xiao-Rong Wu
Hong Xu
Hideyuki Yamamoto
Junn Yanagisawa

Research Assistants
Donara Abramian
Kimberlee J. Dahlin
Christina K. Galang

John Grzesiak
Hiroko Kobayashi
Xiao-Hong Lin
Thomas D. Manes
Jason Miller
Richard Mitchell
Sonoko Narisawa
David P. Schranck
Dianne L. Souza
Sheng-Qi Wang
Tristan Williams
Grace Wood

Research Associates
Liliane A. Dickinson
Ruo-Pan Huang
Shinichi Kudo
Akiko Nishiyama
Matthew J. Schibler
Kathy Soderberg
Jie-Xin Wu

Other Staff
Anders Aspber
Sharon Bodrug
Peter Christmas
Lee Fortunato
Marion Lammertz
Bridget Lollo
Andrew Magnet
Jun Nakayama
Anthony Stevens
Kristina Vuori
Zhuohua Zhang

BOARD OF TRUSTEES

Jim Allen
HST
San Diego, California

Ronald P. Bird
San Diego National Bank
San Diego, California

Malin Burnham, Chairman
John Burnham & Company
San Diego, California

Ernest E. Chipman
La Jolla, California

Raymond V. Dittamore
Ernst & Young
San Diego, California

Catherine Z. Dorn
Denver, Colorado

M. Wainwright Fishburn, Jr.
Cooley Godward Castro Huddleson &
Tatum
San Diego, California

Walter Fitch, III
La Jolla, California

Kenneth H. Golden
Kenneth H. Golden Company
San Diego, California

Elizabeth L. Knox
La Jolla, California

William J. McGill, Ph.D.
University of California at San Diego
La Jolla, California

Thomas A. Page
San Diego Gas & Electric
San Diego, California

Robert A. Rist
Coldwell Banker Residential Affiliates,
Inc.
Mission Viejo, California

Kenneth B. Roath
Healthcare Property Investors, Inc.
Los Angeles, California

Eugene Roberts, Ph.D.
City of Hope National Medical Center
Duarte, California

Edmund H. Shea, Jr.
J.F. Shea Co., Inc.
Walnut, California

Armi K. Williams
La Jolla, California

Scott N. Wolfe, Esq.
Latham & Watkins
San Diego, California

Erkki Ruoslahti, M.D.
President & Chief Executive Officer
La Jolla Cancer Research Foundation
La Jolla, California

Louis R. Coffman
La Jolla Cancer Research Foundation
La Jolla, California

William H. Fishman, Ph.D., M.D. hc
President Emeritus
La Jolla Cancer Research Foundation
La Jolla, California

Special Board Appointments
Theodor H. Heinrichs
Honorary Trustee
San Rafael, California

Winifred Deming
Honorary Trustee
La Jolla, California

Capt. Armistead B. Smith, Jr., USN (Ret.)
Ex officio member Board of Trustees
La Jolla, California

APPENDIX C

PROGRAMS OF LJCRF SYMPOSIA (1981-1994)

1981:   Cellular Differentiation at the Molecular Level

Eileen Adamson	Epidermal Growth Factor Receptors on Embryonal Cells
Elwood Linney	Gene Expression in Teratocarcinomas
Mario Capecchi	Transformation by Direct Nuclear Injection of DNA
Geoffrey Cooper	Analysis of Cellular Transformation by Transfection
Richard Maki	The Role of DNA Rearrangement and Alternative RNA Processing in the Expression of Immunoglobulin Delta Genes
Randolf Wall	Post-Transcriptional Control of Immunoglobulin Gene Expression
William Raschke	Regulation of Immunoglobulin Expression

1982:   The Biology of Metastasis

G. Barry Pierce	Embryonic Control of Malignancy
Erkki Ruoslahti	Fibronectin and Other Basement Membrane Components: Structure-Function Relationships
Charles Birdwell	Ultrastructure of Endothelial Cell Extracellular Matrix
Denis Gospodarowicz	Extracellular Matrices and Growth Factors in Control of Cell Proliferation
Garth Nicolson	Viral and Oncofetal Antigens in Lymphoma Metastasis to Specific Sites
Lance Liotta	Interaction of Metastatic Cells with Basement Membranes
Everett Sugarbaker	Some Clinical Characteristics of Metastasis in Man

1983:   Are Oncogenes Oncodevelopmental Genes?

J. Michael Bishop	Retroviruses and Cellular Oncogenes
Elwood Linney	Enhancing Sequences in Gene Expression
Tony Hunter	Mechanisms of Cellular Transformation by Viral Oncogenes
Owen Witte	The Abelson Oncogene Interaction with Early Stages of the Murine B Cell Lineage
Mariano Barbacid	Transforming Genes in Human Tumors

Robert A. Weinberg   Oncogenes and Human Tumor Cells

1984:   Cytoskeletal Proteins in Development and Malignancy

Elias Lazarides   Establishment of Membrane - Cytoskeletal
                        Domains in Development: Spectrin as a
                        Model System
Robert G. Oshima   Endodermal Intermediate Filament Protein
                        Expression in Embryos and
                        Teratocarcinoma Cells
Elain V. Fuchs   Differential Expression and Structure
                        of Keratins
Bill R. Brinkley   Microtubule Organizing Centers in Normal and
                        Neoplastic Cells: Recognition of Tubulin
                        Assembly and Distribution
S. Jonathan Singer   Cytoskeletal Interactions in Normal
                        and Malignant Cells
Keith R. Porter   Cytoplasmic Matrix in Normal and
                        Malignant Cells
Ismo Virtanen   Expression of Intermediate Filaments in
                        Developing and Adult Tissues and in Tumors

1985:   Gene Transfer

Inder M. Verma   Gene Transfer Via Retroviral Vectors
Geoffrey Wahl   Regions of Eukaryotic Chromosomes
                        Associated with High Frequency Gene
                        Amplification Revealed by Gene Transfer
Leroy Hood   The T-Cell Receptor and Other Receptors that
                        Regulate the Vertebrate Immune Response
Richard Maki   Molecular and Immunological Aspects of Ia
                        Gene Expression
Richard D. Palmiter   Expression of Genes Introduced into Mice
Gerald M. Rubin   Gene Transfer in Drosophila

1986:   Signaling at the Cell Surface

Michael D. Waterfield   The EGF Receptor: Attempts to Understand
                        Normal and Abnormal Signal Transduction
Harold L. Moses   Transforming Growth Factors: An
                        Indirect Mitogen and a Growth Inhibitor
Robert D. Rosenberg   Heparin-Like Molecules and Cell Growth
                        Regulation
Erkki Ruoslahti   Molecular Anatomy of a Cell Surface
                        Recognition System
Silvio S. Varon   Neurotrophic Factors *In Vitro* and *In Vivo*
Per Peterson   Human MHC Antigens

1987:   Steroid Hormone Receptors, Gene Regulation, and Cancer

Bert O'Malley	Steroid Receptors, Transcription Factors, and Gene Expression
Ron Evans	Steroid and Thyroid Hormone Receptors: A Superfamily of Regulatory Proteins
Michael Karin	Regulation of Gene Expression by Hormone-Responsive and Tissue-Specific Trans-acting Factors
Magnus Pfahl	Steroid Hormone Receptors and Promoter Activation
Gordon Ringold	Hormone Control of Cell Differentiation
Bernd Groner	Cellular Responses to the Activation of Oncogenes
Marc E. Lippman	Estrogenic control of Growth Factor Production by Human Breast Cancer

1988:   Adhesive Interactions in Cell Migration and Morphogenesis

Gerald Edelman	Adhesion Molecules in the Regulation of Animal Form and Tissue Pattern
Jean-Paul Thiery	Adhesion Modes in Embryonic Cell Motility and in Epithelial-Mesenchymal Conversion
David Bentley	Pathfinding by Growth Cones of Peripheral Pioneer Neurons in an Insect Embryo
Eva Engvall	Unique and Ubiquitous Basement Membrane Components: Effects on Cells and Expression During Development
Samuel Barondes	Endogenous Soluble Lectins: Functions in Morphogenesis and Extracellular Matrix
Irving Weissman	Homing and Differentiation of Hematolymphoid Cells

1989:   Nuclear Proteins as Gene Regulators in Development and Oncogenesis

Pierre Chambon	Nuclear Receptors as Inducible Transcription Enhancers
Peter Vogt	Jun - Transcriptional Factor and Oncogene
Magnus Pfahl	Do Nuclear Receptors Cross Talk?
Patrick O'Farrell	Homeodomain Proteins are Transcriptional Regulators Related by Functional as well as Sequence Homologies
Ronald Evans	Molecular Genetics of Steroid and Thyroid Hormone Receptors
Winship Herr	Differential Activation of Transcription by the Ubiquitous and Cell Specific Transcription Factors Oct-1 and Oct-2

Michael Karin — Transacting Factors Controlling Cellular Proliferation and Differentiation: AP-1 and GHF-1

1990: Gene Regulation in Mammalian Development

Roger Pedersen — Differentiation and Fate in the Extra-embryonic Lineages of Mouse Embryos
Sidney Strickland — Activation of Maternal mRNA During Meiosis
Eileen Adamson — Transcription Factor Responses to Retinoic Acid in Embryonal Carcinoma Cells
Peter Gruss — Murine Developmental Control Genes
Rudolf Jaenisch — Mutations in Transgenic Mice
Janet Rossant — Identification and Mutation of Genes Involved in Mouse Development
Oliver Smithies — The Drell Lecture - Altering Genes in Animals

1991: Molecular Mechanisms of Tumor Growth and Suppression

Ray White — Characterization of the Gene for Neurofibromatosis Type I
Stephen H. Friend — Cancer Risks from Germ-Line Mutations in Tumor Suppressor Genes
Tony Hunter — Protein Phosphorylation in the Cell Cycle and Growth Control
Douglas R. Lowy — Transformation by Ras and Other Non-Nuclear Oncoproteins
Lewis T. Williams — Signal Transduction by the PDGF and FGF Receptors
Frank McCormick — Regulation of Ras Proteins by GTPase Activating Proteins
Henry R. Bourne — G Protein Oncogenes

1992: Hematopoiesis in Normal and Abnormal Development

Erkki Ruoslahti — Opening Remarks
Stuart H. Orkin — Development of the Erythroid Lineage *In Vivo* and *In Vitro*
Harvey F. Lodish — The Erythropoietin and TGF-ß Receptors: Signal Transduction and Tumorigenesis
E. Richard Stanley — Biology and Action of Colony Stimulating Factor-1
Hitoshi Sakano — Somatic DNA Rearrangement in the Immune and Central Nervous Systems
Michiko N. Fukuda — HEMPAS: Genetic Anemia Caused by Defective Glycosylation
Steven D. Rosen — L-Selectin: A Lectin-Like Leukocyte Adhesion Protein

Irving L. Weissman Hematopoietic Stem Cells and Lymphocyte
         Development

1993: Molecular Control of Neural Development

Masatoshi Takeichi Molecular Basis of Specific Cell-Cell Adhesion
         and Multicellular Organization
Barbara Ranscht   Cell Adhesion Molecules During Axon Growth
         and Patterning
Corey Goodman   Genetic Analysis of Pathway and Target
         Recognition During Neuronal Development in
         Drosophila
Uel J. McMahan   The Role of Agrin in Synaptogenesis
Gerald M. Rubin   The Signal Transduction Pathway Initiated by
         Activation of the Sevenless Tyrosine Kinase
         Receptor
Andy McMahon   Wnt-gene Signaling is Essential for Regulation
         of Axial Development and CNS Patterning in
         Mouse Development
George Yancopoulos Neurotrophic Factors and How They Work
Susumu Tonegawa Use of the Gene Knock Out Technique for the
         Analysis of Mammalian Learning

1994: Cell Differentiation: models and applications

Mina J. Bissell   Signal Transduction from Extracellular Matrix:
         Implications for Development and Breast
         Cancer
Ruth Sager   Down Regulation of Genes with Tumor
         Suppressing Activity in Breast Cancer
José Luis Millán   Using Immortalized Germ Cells to Study
         Meiosis and Spermatogenesis in Vitro
Beatrice Mintz   Growth Factors in Transgenic Mouse Models
         of Melanoma
Ron McKay   Mammalian Neuronal Stem Cells
Helen M. Blau   Myoblast Mediated Gene Therapy: A Novel
         Form of Drug Delivery
Richard C. Mulligan Gene Therapy for Diseases Affecting
         Hematopoietic Cells
Ernest Beutler   Transplantation of Stem Cells in Humans:
         Problems and Promise

APPENDIX D

1989 ALKALINE PHOSPHATASE SYMPOSIUM
TO HONOR THE CAREER OF
WILLIAM H. FISHMAN, PH.D., M.D. hc
—organized by José L. Millán

Session I: Structure of AP Genes

Harry Harris	Keynote lecture: The Human Alkaline Phosphatases: What We Know and What We Don't Know
José Luis Millán	Oncodevelopmental Expression of Alkaline Phosphatase Genes: Going from Structure to Function
Brian Knoll	Comparative and Functional Analysis of Human Alkaline Phosphatase Genes
Gideon A. Rodan	Rat Alkaline Phosphatases: Cloning, Expression and Regulation on Osteoblastic Cells
Kazuya Higashino	Molecular Cloning and Sequence Analysis of the Kasahara Isoenzyme

Session II: Allelic Polymorphism in AP Genes

Howard H. Sussman	Restriction Fragment Length Polymorphism of the Human Placental Alkaline Phosphatase Gene
Derek Tucker*	Molecular Genetic Analysis of the Human Placental Alkaline Phosphatase Gene and Related Sequences
Tsugikazu Komoda	Allelic and Ectopic Polymorphisms of Human Placental Alkaline Phosphatases
Lars Beckman	Correlation Between Restriction Fragment Length Polymorphism and Electrophoretic Types of Human Placental Alkaline Phosphatase

*Passed away Dec. 1st, 1988. Ian Campbell presented Derek's lecture.

Session III: Structural-Functional Studies on AP

Harold W. Wyckoff	Three-Dimensional Structure of Alkaline Phosphatases
Janusz M. Sowadski	Structural Relationships in the Alkaline Phosphatase Family

Session IV: Membrane Anchoring Mechanisms of Alkaline Phosphatases

Carole A. Bailey	Requirements for the Processing of Nascent Placental Alkaline Phosphatase to Its Mature Form
Yukio Ikehara	Membrane-Anchoring Mechanism of Human Placental Alkaline Phosphatase
Robert A. Stinson	Incorporation of Human Alkaline Phosphatase into Liposomes by Phosphatidylinositol Phospholipase C
Martin G. Low	Degradation of the Phosphatidylinositol Anchor of Alkaline Phosphatase by Endogenous Enzymes
M. Edward Medof	Structural Modulations of the Glycosylinositol Phospholipid (GPL) Anchor of Placental Alkaline Phosphatase (PLAP)

Session V: Clinical Significance of AP Isozyme Determinations

Donald W. Moss	Pathological and Diagnostic Aspects of Multiple Forms of Alkaline Phosphatase in Serum
Michael P. Whyte	Alkaline Phosphatase: Physiologic Role Explored in Hypophosphatasia
Patricia M. Crofton	A Paediatric Focus on Alkaline Phosphatase Isoenzyme Problems
John Griffith	The Regan Isozyme - Revisited Alternate Origin to the Placental Source
David Brocklehurst	The Inverse Relationship Between Intestinal and the Particulate Form of Alkaline Phosphatase in Human Hepatic Disease

Session VI: AP Expression in Cell Cultures

Janice Y. Chou	Human Choriocarcinoma Cells Express the Germ-Cell Alkaline Phosphatase Gene
David H. Alper	Pathways of Alkaline Phosphatase Secretion from Rat Enterocytes
Young S. Kim	Alkaline Phosphatase Expression During Differentiation in Colon Cancer Cells
William H. Fishman	Forty Years in the Land of Phosphatases

Session VII: Alkaline Phosphatases in Early Embryogenesis

Carol A. Ziomek	Stage-Specific Expression of a Heat-Stable Alkaline Phosphatase in Preimplantation Mouse Embryos
Gilbert A. Schultz	Alkaline Phosphatase of Mouse Embryonal Carcinoma Cells and Preimplantation Embryos

| Malcom A. Steinberg | Is Alkaline Phosphatase Involved in Guiding Embryonal Cell Migrations? |

Session VIII: Alkaline Phosphatases as Tumor Markers

Etienne Nouwen	Pulmonary Heat-Stable Alkaline Phosphatase in Man and Primates. Expression and Release
J. Hustin	The Ontogenesis of Placental Alkaline Phosphatase Expression. Extension to Various Gonadal Pathologies
Shiro Nozawa	Serum PLAP Levels in Gynaecological Malignancies

Session IX: Alkaline Phosphatases in Testicular Tumors

Kiyoshi Koshida	Heterogeneity of PLAP in Seminomas
Kazuyuki Hirano	Purification and Properties of Placental-Like and Tissue-Unspecific Alkaline Phosphatases in Seminoma Tissue
Bent Norgaard-Pedersen	Clinical Significance of AFP, HCG and PLAP in 272 Seminoma Patients. A Prospective Study
Peter M. Johnson	Application of Monoclonal Antibodies and PLAP-cDNA to Study the Expression of PLAP and PLAP-Like Isozymes

Session X: Immunolocalization of AP Producing Tumors

| Kjell Nustad | *In Vivo* Evaluation of Radiolabelled Anti-PLAP Antibodies with Cells or Antigen-Coated Particles in Diffusion Chambers |
| Torgny Stigbrand | Radioimmunolocalization and Radioimmunotherapy Using Anti-PLAP Monoclonal Antibodies |

AUTHORS, COLLABORATORS, 1942-1989.

A ARTOM, C., ANLYAN, A.J., ARTENSTEIN, M., ASHMORE, J., ANTISS, C., ABRAHAM, R, ANGELLIS, D., AVIOLI, L.V.

B BERNFELD, P., BIGELOW, R., BONNER, C.D., BRANCHE, G., BAKER, J.R., BENJAMIN, G., BORGES, P.R.F.

C COHN, M., CONTI, P., CUBELLIS, A., COOK, W.B., CLARKE, B.G., CHENEY, M., CHIN, F., CLOSE, V.A., COTE, R.A., CANTOR, F., CLARK, L.A., CHANG, C.-H.

D DART, R.M., DAVIDSON, H., DIMITRAKIS, H., DELELLIS,R., DORSAY, R.H., DAS, I., DRISCOLL, S.G., DOELLGAST, G.J., DEMPO, K., DESMOND, W.

E ELLIOTT, K.A.C.

F FISHMAN, L., FARMELANT, M., FIALKOW, P.J., FRIEDEN, E.H., FARRON-FURSTENSTAHL, F.

G GOVIER, W., GORDON, E., GREEN, S., GRIMALDI, R., GOLDMAN, S.S., GHOSH, N.K., GIOVANNIELLO, T.J., GUZEK, D.T., GANDBHIR, L.

H HUGGINS, C., HOMBURGER, F., HEW, H., HAYASHI, M., HABLANIAN, A., HARPER, A.A., HARRIS, F., HIROHATA, I., HABIB, H., HANFORD, W.C.

I INGLIS, N.R., IDE, H., IBSEN, K., IINO, S.

J JEMMERSON, R.

K KREISHER, J.H., KRANT, M.J., KATO, K., KOTOWITZ, L., KIRLEY, S., KELLY, J.P.W., KOTTEL, R.H., KRISHNASWAMY, P.R., KURIHARA, S., KANO, S., KLIER, F.G.

L LEVEEN, H.H., LERNER, F., LEADBETTER, W.F., LIPKIND, J.B., LADUE, K.T., LINSCHEER, W.G., LIN, C.-W., LITTLEFIELD, J.W., LANGE, P.H.

M MOREHEAD, R.P., MARKUS, R.L., MCGOWAN, J., MITCHELL JR., G.W., MAHLER, R., MATHUR, G.P., MANNING, J.P., MALAGELADA, J.R., MARSH, C.A., MIYAYAMA, H., MEMOLI, V., MILLAN, J.L.

N NISSELBAUM, J.S., NIGAM, V.N., NAKAHARA, W., NAKAJIMA, Y., NATHANSON, L., NISHIYAMA, T., NAPOLI, A.D., NOZAWA, S.

O ODELL, L.D., ORCUTT, M.L., OHTA, H.

P PAGE, O.C., PFEIFFER, P.H., PETTENGILL, O.S., PLAUT, A.G., PATTERSON, J.F., PIRNIK, M.

Q

R ROMSEY, E., RIOTTON, G., ROBINSON, M.J., REIF, A., RUSTIGIAN, R., RUFO, M., RAAM, S., RULE, A., RUOSLAHTI, E.

S SHORR, E., SPRINGER, B., SMITH, M., SIE, H.-G., STOLBACH, L.L., SAWYER, D., SMITH, R.E., SHIRAHAMA, T., SHARKEY, L.J., SASAKI, M., SINGER, R., SOLOMON, R., SELL, S., STIGBRAND, T STAHL, P.D., SHAH, N.

T TALALAY, P., THOMPSON, D.B., TAKEUCHI, T., TSUKAMOTO, H., TOKUMITSU, S. & K., TAKEYA, M.

U UDAGAWA, Y.

V VAITUKAITIS, J., VESSELLA, R.-L.

W WAYNE, A., WOTIZ, H., WAKABAYASHI, M., WATANABE, K., WENTWORTH, M.A., WARSHAW, J.B., WHYTE, M.P.

X

Y YORSHIS, E., YUKI, H.

Z

REFERENCES

1. Pierre Berton "The Promised Land" A Penguin Books Canada, McClelland & Stewart Book, 1984.

2. Henry Taube-Nobel Laureate in Chemistry, 1983.

3. Fishman, W.H. The application of the ether-partitioning method to metabolic studies on <u>clostridium</u> <u>acetobutylicum</u>. <u>Thesis</u>, University of Toronto, 1939.

4. Fishman, W.H. Studies on ß-glucuronidase. I. A method of preparation and purification. <u>J. Biol. Chem.</u> <u>127</u>:367-373, 1939.

5. Fishman, W.H. Studies on ß-glucuronidase. II. Factors controlling the initial velocity of hydrolysis of some conjugated glucuronides. <u>J. Biol. Chem.</u> <u>131</u>:225-232, 1939.

6. Fishman, W.H. Studies on ß-glucuronidase. III. The increase in ß-glucuronidase activity of mammalian tissues induced by feeding glucuronidogenic substances. <u>J. Biol. Chem.</u> <u>136</u>:229-236, 1940.

7. The Fishman Tissue Minihomogenizer. <u>Thesis</u>, University of Toronto, 1939.

8. Fishman, L., Miyayama, H., Driscoll, S., and Fishman, W.H. Developmental phase-specific alkaline phosphatase isoenzymes of human placenta and their occurrence in human cancer. <u>Cancer Res.</u> <u>367</u>:2268-2273, 1976.

9. Fishman, L. Acrylamide disc gel electrophoresis of alkaline phosphatase of human tissues, serum and ascites fluid using Triton X-100 in the sample and the gel matrix. <u>Biochem. Med.</u> <u>9</u>:309-315, 1974.

10. Fishman, W.H., and Fishman, L. The elevation of uterine ß-glucuronidase activity by estrogenic hormones. <u>J. Biol. Chem.</u> <u>152</u>:487-488, 1944.

11. Fishman, W.H., and Cohn, M. A comparative study of acetylation in vivo of phenylaminobutyric acid with p-aminobenzoic acid and sulfanilamide. <u>J. Biol. Chem.</u> <u>148</u>:619-626, 1943.

12. Artom, C., and Fishman, W.H. The relation of the diet to the composition of tissue phospholipids. I. The normal composition of liver and muscle lipids of the rat, with a note on the analytical procedures. <u>J. Biol. Chem.</u> <u>148</u>:405-414, 1943.

13. Fishman, W.H., and Artom, C. Serine injury. J. Biol. Chem. 145:345-346, 1942.

14. Talalay, P., Fishman, W.H., and Huggins, C. Chromogenic substrates. II. Phenolphthalein glucuronic acid as substrate for the assay of glucuronidase activity. J. Biol. Chem. 166:757-772, 1946.

15. Fishman, W.H., and Anlyan, A.J. The presence of high ß-glucuronidase activity in cancer tissue. J. Biol. Chem. 169:449-450, 1947.

16. Warburg, O. Ueber den Stoffwechsel der Tumoren, Berlin; Springer, 1926.

17. Pettengill, O.S., and Fishman, W.H. The preparation and purification of ß-glucuronidase from mouse liver, kidney and urine. J. Biol. Chem. 237:24-28, 1962.

18. Pettengill, O.S., and Fishman, W.H. Influence of testosterone on glycine incorporation into mouse kidney ß-glucuronidase. Exp. Cell Research 28:248-253, 1962.

19. Li, M.C., Hertz, R., and Spencer, D.B. Effect of methotrexate therapy upon choriocarcinoma and chorioadenoma. Proc. Soc. Exp. Biol. & Med. 93:361-366, 1956.

20. Stolbach, L., Krant, M.J., and Fishman, W.H. Ectopic production of an alkaline phosphatase isoenzyme in patients with cancer. New Eng. J. Med. 281:757-762, 1969.

21. Fishman, W.H., Goldman, S., and DeLellis, R. Dual localization of ß-glucuronidase in endoplasmic reticulum and in lysosomes. Nature 213:457-460, 1967.

22. Fialkow, P.J., and Fishman, W.H. Studies on a liver activator of ß-glucuronidase. J. Biol. Chem. 236:2169-2171, 1961.

23. Abdul-Fadl, M.A.M., and King, E.J. Properties of acid phosphatase of erythrocytes and of human prostate gland. Biochem. J. 45:51-60, 1949.

24. Fishman, W.H., and Lerner, F. A method for estimating serum acid phosphatase of prostatic origin. J. Biol. Chem. 200:89-97, 1953.

25. Fishman, W.H., Kasdon, C.S., and Homburger, F. ß-glucuronidase studies in women. I. Observations in 500 non-pregnant non-cancerous subjects. J. Am. Med. Assoc. 143:350-354, 1950.

26. Kasdon, S.C., Fishman, W.H., and Homburger, F. ß-glucuronidase studies in women. II. Cancer of the cervix uteri. J. Am. Med. Assoc. 144:892-896, 1950.

27. Bernfeld, P., and Fishman, W.H. ß-glucuronidase. I. Purification of calf liver spleen ß-glucuronidase. J. Biol. Chem. 202:757-762, 1953.

28. Bernfeld, P., Nisselbaum, J.S., and Fishman, W.H. ß-glucuronidase. II. Purification of calf liver ß-glucuronidase. J. Biol. Chem. 202:763-769, 1953.

29. Fishman, W.H., Dart, R.M., Bonner, C.D., Leadbetter, W.F., Lerner, F., and Homburger, F. A new method for estimating serum acid phosphatase of prostatic origin applied to the clinical investigation of cancer of the prostate. J. Clin. Inv. 32:1034-1044, 1953.

30. Fishman, W.H., Green, S., and Inglis, N. L-phenylalanine: an organ-specific, stereospecific inhibitor of human intestinal alkaline phosphatase (EC 3.1.3.1), Nature 198:685-686, 1963.

31. Green, S., Anstiss, C.L., and Fishman, W.H. Automated differential isoenzyme analysis. II. The fractionation of serum alkaline phosphatases into "liver", "intestinal" and "other" components. Enzymologia 41:9-26, 1971.

32. Neale, F.C., Cubb, J.S., Hotchkiss, D., and Posen, S. Heat stability of human placental alkaline phosphatase. J. Clin. Path. 18:359-363, 1965.

33. Fishman, W.H., Inglis, N.R., Stolbach, L.L., and Krant, M.J. A serum alkaline phosphatase isoenzyme of human neoplastic cell origin. Cancer Res. 28:150-154, 1968.

34. Nathanson, L., and Fishman, W.H. New observations on the Regan isoenzyme of alkaline phosphatase in cancer patients. Cancer 27:1388-1397, 1971.

35. Lange, P.H., Millán, J.L., Stigbrand, T., Vesella, R.G., Ruoslahti, E. and Fishman, W.H. Placental alkaline phosphatase as a tumor marker for seminoma. Cancer Res. 3244-3247, 1982.

36. Epenetos, A.A., Carr, D., Johnson, P.M., Bodner, W.F., and Lavender, J.P. Antibody-guided radiolocalization of tumors in patients with testicular or ovarian cancer using two radioiodinated monoclonal antibodies to placental alkaline phosphatase. Br. J. Radiol. 59:117-125, 1986

37. Abelev, G.I. Alpha-fetoprotein in ontogenesis and its association with malignant tumors. Adv. Cancer Res. 14:295-358, 1971.

38. Tatarinov, Y.S. Detection of embryo-specific α-globulin in the blood sera of a patient with primary liver tumor. Vopr. Med. Khim. 10:90-91, 1964.

39. Gold, P., and Freedman, S.O. Demonstration of tumor-specific antigens in human colonic carcinomata by immunological tolerance and absorption techniques. J. Expl. Med. 121:439-462, 1965.

40. Hatzfeld, A., Weber, A., and Schapira, F. Biochemical and immunological studies of some carcinofetal enzymes. Ann. N.Y. Acad. Sci. 259:287-297, 1975.

41. Weinhouse, S. Glycolysis, respiration and anomalous gene expression in experimental hepatomas. G.H.A. Clowes memorial lecture. Cancer Res. 32:2007-2016, 1972.

42. Hirai, H. and Alpert, E. Carcinofetal Proteins: Biology and Chemistry. Ann. N.Y. Acad. Sci. 259:1-452, 1975

43. Fishman, W.H., and Sell, S. Regulation of gene expression in development and neoplasia - San Diego conference on oncodevelopmental gene expression: May 29 to June 1, 1976. Cancer Research 36:4205-4330, 1976.

44. Fishman, W.H., and Sell, S. (eds.) ONCO-DEVELOPMENTAL GENE EXPRESSION. Academic Press, Inc. (publ.), New York, 1-781, 1976.

45. Iino, S., and Fishman, L. The effects of sucrose and other carbohydrates on human alkaline phosphatase isoenzyme activity. Clin. Chim. Acta. 92:197-207, 1979.

46. Millán, J.L. Third Alkaline Phosphatase Symposium. Clin. Chim. Acta. 186:125-320, 1990.

47. Warburg, O. The Metabolism of Tumors, London, Arnold Constable, 1930.

48. Pitot, H. Fundamentals of Oncology. Marcel Dekker, Inc., New York, Publisher 1986

49. Greenstein, J.P. Biochemistry of Cancer. Edition 2, New York, Academic Press, Inc., Publisher, 1954.

50. Miller, J.A., and Miller, E.C. The carcinogenic aminoazodyes. Adv. Cancer Res. 1:339-96, 1953.

51. Pierce, G.B. Teratocarcinoma: model for a developmental concept of cancer. Curr. Topics Dev. Biol. 2:223-246, 1967.

52. Mintz, B., and Illmensee, K. Normal genetically mosaic mice produced from malignant teratocarcinoma cells. Proc. Natl. Acad. Sci. U.S.A. 72:3585-3589, 1975.

53. Fishman, W.H. Perspectives on alkaline phosphatase isoenzymes. Am. J. Med. 56:617-650, 1974.

54. Ruoslahti, E., and Terry, W.D. α-Fetoprotein and serum albumin show sequence homology. Nature 260:804-805, 1976.

55. Ruoslahti, E., and Engvall, E. Immunological crossreaction between alpha-fetoprotein and albumin. Proc. Natl. Acad. Sci. 73:4641-4644, 1976.

56. Engvall, E. Pregnancy-specific ß-1-glycoprotein (SP₁). Purification and partial characterization. Oncodevelopmental Biol. and Med. 1: 113-122, 1980.

57. Hammerstrom, S., Engvall, E., Johansson, B.G., Svenson, S., Sundblad, G., and Goldstein, I.J. Nature of the tumor-associated determinant(s) of carcino-embryonic antigen (CEA). Proc. Natl. Acad. Sci. 72: 1528-1532, 1975.

58. Engvall, E., and Perlmann, D. Enzyme-linked immunosorbent assay, ELISA. Quantitation assay of immunoglobulin G. Immunochem. 8:871-874, 1971.

59. Engvall, E. and Ruoslahti, E. Binding of soluble form of fibroblast surface protein, fibronectin, to collagen. Int. J. Cancer 20:1-5, 1977.

60. Pierschbacher, M., Ruoslahti, E., Sundelin, J., Lind, P., and Peterson, P.A. Cell attachment domain of fibronectin—Determination of the primary structure. J. Biol. Chem. 257:9593-9597, 1982.

61. Fishman, W.H. The 1993 ISOBM ABBOTT AWARD. Enzymes, Tumor Markers and Oncodevelopmental Biology. Tumor Biology. 16:394-402, 1995.

INDEX

ORDER FORM

**The La Jolla Cancer Research Foundation -
The Miracle on Torrey Pines Mesa.**
Price: $18.50*

No. of copies: _____

Ship to

Name: _____

Address: _____

City: _____

State: _____ Zip code: _____

Telephone #: _____

Payment method:

☐ Check

Credit Card:

☐ Visa   ☐ M.C.

Name on Card: _____

Card #: _____ Exp. Date: _____

Price includes sales tax and shipping

Please mail payment to:
**La Jolla Cancer Research Foundation
10901 N. Torrey Pines Rd.
La Jolla, CA 92037**

ORDER FORM

The La Jolla Cancer Research Foundation -
The Miracle on Torrey Pines Mesa.
Price: $18.50*

No. of copies: _____

Ship to

Name: _____

Address: _____

City: _____

State: _____ Zip code: _____

Telephone #: _____

Payment method:

☐ Check

Credit Card:

☐ Visa   ☐ M.C.

Name on Card: _____

Card #: _____ Exp. Date: _____

Price includes sales tax and shipping

Please mail payment to:
La Jolla Cancer Research Foundation
10901 N. Torrey Pines Rd.
La Jolla, CA 92037